A Special Issue of
Cognition & Emotion

Emotional Memory Failures

Edited by

Ineke Wessel
University of Groningen,
The Netherlands

and

Daniel B. Wright
University of Sussex, UK

Psychology Press
Taylor & Francis Group
HOVE AND NEW YORK

First published in 2004 by Psychology Press Ltd
27 Church Road, Hove, East Sussex, BN3 2FA

Simultaneously published in the USA and Canada
by Taylor & Francis Inc
711 Third Avenue, New York, NY 10017

First issued in paperback 2015

Psychology Press is an imprint of the Taylor and Francis Group, an informa business

British Library Cataloguing in Publication Data
A catalogue record for this book is available from the British Library

ISBN 13: 978-1-138-88327-7 (pbk)
ISBN 13: 978-1-84169-931-8 (hbk)

ISSN 0269-9931

Typeset by DP Photosetting, Aylesbury, Bucks

This publication has been produced with paper manufactured to strict environmental standards and with pulp derived from sustainable forests.

Contents*

*This book is also a special issue of the journal *Cognition & Emotion*, and forms issue 4 of Volume 18 (2004). The page numbers are taken from the journal and so begin with p. 449.

COGNITION AND EMOTION, 2004, *18* (4), 449–455

Emotional memory failures: On forgetting and reconstructing emotional experiences

Ineke Wessel
University of Groningen, The Netherlands

Daniel B. Wright
University of Sussex, Brighton, UK

It was dubbed the *memory wars*. Psychology and psychiatry were showing their dirty laundry in full view of the courts, the media, and heated debates at conferences and workshops (McNally, 2003). As memory researchers we felt a sense of importance. Instead of writing articles just for fellow academics, we were addressing critical questions about *recovered memories* that were of interest to the readers of Time and Newsweek. The term "recovered memories" referred to recollections of trauma (usually sexual abuse) that emerged in individuals who previously thought that their life had been uneventful. The debate was between those who believed that many of the memories were created in people's imagination (sometimes with guidance from mental health professionals) and those who believed that many of the memories were previously inaccessible, but basically accurate, accounts of past events. There are two distinct questions here. Can false memories for entire events be created in people's memories? And, what happens to memories of true emotional events?

The first wave of memory research addressed the first question. Loftus (e.g., 1997) and others showed that memories for entire events could be added to people's autobiography. While these researchers were constrained by research ethics committees not to try to add highly emotive events to people's memories, others did not have these constraints. As shown in high profile court cases, like those against mental health professionals Bennett Braun and Judith Peterson, highly emotive events, like satanic ritual abuse, can be added to people's memories. Even those who argue that trauma often leads to psychogenic amnesia (through repression, dissociation, etc.) recognise that false memories can be implanted into people's memories (Ross, 2001). Of course showing that

Correspondence should be addressed to Ineke Wessel, Department of Clinical and Developmental Psychology, University of Groningen, Grote Kruisstraat 2–1, 9712 TS Groningen, The Netherlands; e-mail: I.Wessel@ppsw.rug.nl

http://www.tandf.co.uk/journals/pp/02699931.html DOI:10.1080/02699930341000383

false memories can be created does not show that all recovered memories are false. It only shows that some may be false.

The second question, how emotional events are remembered, is addressed in this Special Issue. It is clear that much trauma exists: Every day many people become victims of war, disasters, abuse, etc. Many experimental psychologists have learned how to appreciate the value of clinical case studies. In addition, field studies of trauma and memory are informative. For example, anthropologist Judith Zur (1998) studied the war widows in El Quiché, Guatemala. In an Orwellian fashion, the widows were to forget their memories, not to commemorate the dead, and even to remarry. The resulting memories show elements of both recovery, ''the event triggered memories which previously had not seemed to exist at all'' (p. 167), and distortion, ''women incorporate into their own memories the details of other people's memories, even those details they may have denied earlier'' (p. 171).

While case studies and field research can show how psychological phenomena manifest themselves in the frontline of the memory wars, they lack the control that many psychologists want in order to understand the causal mechanisms involved. The papers in this Special Issue examine how people remember emotional material with the aim of teasing apart some of the causal mechanisms. The papers ask what mechanisms underlie forgetting of emotive events, if certain people process memories for emotive events differently, and if memory distortions can be shown for major events.

Forgetting of emotional material

Over the past decade, the study of mechanisms underlying forgetting has become increasingly popular. The retrieval-induced forgetting (RIF; Anderson, Bjork, & Bjork, 1994) paradigm has been used particularly often, with a variety of materials (e.g., words, visuospatial objects, mock crimes, personality traits, see Levy & Anderson, 2002 for an overview). In their current contribution, Barnier, Hung, and Conway extend these findings to memories of personally experienced events. They asked their participants to generate positive, negative, and neutral autobiographical memories. Next, they used this material in a basic RIF procedure. That is, in a retrieval practice phase, participants repeatedly retrieved and elaborated upon only a selection of the memories (but in all affective valence categories). Unsurprisingly, a later recall test rendered good performance for these practised items. However, recall of items that were related to the practised items was impaired relative to a baseline of unrelated items. This was the case for memories in all affective categories. Barnier et al.'s findings are important in that they are the first to report RIF for highly complex and emotional memories.

In RIF, forgetting is more or less a by-product of extensively rehearsing other related material. What happens if people try their best to wilfully forget emotional experiences? McNally, Clancy, Barrett, and Parker employed a directed forgetting procedure to examine the often-heard claim in the recovered memory debate that survivors of child sexual abuse would be skilled forgetters of trauma-related memories (e.g., Cloitre, 1998). The authors tested participants who reportedly had repressed (i.e., who believed they were abused, but had no memories of it), recovered (i.e., had memories of abuse that were previously forgotten), or continuous (i.e., had memories of abuse that they always remembered) memories and a never-abused control group. McNally and co-workers aimed at finding out whether these groups differed in the extent to which they were able to intentionally forget positive and trauma-related words when instructed to do so. Their findings indicate that overall, less to-be-forgotten than to-be-remembered words were recalled. However, groups did not differ in their forgetting abilities, not for positive and not for trauma-related words. Thus, the claim that people with repressed or recovered memories are better forgetters could not be corroborated.

Do some people forget more easily than others?

Even if people who report that they were molested as a child are not more skilled at forgetting trauma-related material, the question remains whether there are other variables that predict forgetting. Three studies in this issue concentrate on the personality characteristic of repressive coping. Repressive copers (or repressors) are people who do not easily report negative affect, but do react physiologically to emotional stimuli (Myers, 2000). Interestingly, there is evidence that repressors also show a specific memory deficit. For example, Myers, Brewin and Power (1998) found that repressors show more directed forgetting than nonrepressors, but only for negative and not for positive self-referent material. In their current contribution, Myers and Derakshan add two important manipulations to the directed forgetting (DF) procedure of Myers et al.'s earlier study. First, for purpose of manipulating self-referent encoding, participants rated to what extent negative or positive adjectives described either themselves or their peers. Second, participants were led to believe that they were tested under private (alone) or public (under scrutiny of an experimenter) conditions. Myers and Derakshan's results replicate earlier findings that repressors show more directed forgetting than nonrepressors. However, they also found that this effect was specific: It was restricted to negative self-referent words under private testing conditions.

Barnier, Levin, and Maher wondered whether repressors are better than nonrepressors in not thinking of unwanted emotional personal memories. In order to test this, they adapted Wegner's (see Wegner, 1989) well-known thought suppression (TS) paradigm. Rather than not thinking of white bears as in the original paradigm, Barnier and colleagues instructed their participants not to think of an emotional personal memory (about being extremely proud or extremely embarrassed). They found that repressors, compared to nonrepressor control groups, tended to be more successful in avoiding thoughts of the embarrassed event. In contrast, repressive copers showed no suppression advantage for the proud event.

Taken together, the results of these two studies suggest that the mechanism underlying repressors' specific impairment in recalling negative self-referent material should be in the retrieval stage of memory processing. However, on an individual level, these studies are not conclusive that, indeed, differences in retrieval strategy explain differences between repressors and nonrepressors. That is, the DF results of Myers and Derakshan still leave room for an interpretation in terms of differential encoding. Likewise, Barnier, Levin, and Maher's findings are silent about whether successful suppression results in a poorer quality of the target memory. In their contribution, Shane and Peterson set out to disentangle to what extent encoding and retrieval contribute to the specific memory patterns found in repressors. Participants studied positive, negative, and neutral words that were later tested with a free recall test. In addition, they participated in a go/no go task that was designed to differentiate to what extent people allocate processing resources to negative feedback during encoding and retrieval. Shane and Peterson found that defensiveness was associated with less recall of negative words. Note that in contrast with the findings of Myers and Derakshan, these words were not encoded under self-referential conditions. Interestingly, Shane and Peterson's results also suggest that the relation between defensiveness and memory was mediated by the tendency to allocate less processing resources to retrieval of instances of earlier failure. Thus, repressors' tendency to avoid retrieval of negative material may be the most likely candidate to explain their specific recall patterns. Shane and Peterson refer to these recall patterns in terms of self-induced memory distortion: A tendency to distort reality for such varied purposes as mood regulation, justification of goals, maintaining self-concept, etc. It is important to note that this type of distortion refers to a bias (away from negative and towards positive material) rather than incorporating incorrect, nonexisting information into memory. We turn to this latter type of distortion—false memories—next.

Emotion and memory errors

A frequently-heard criticism on false memory studies has been that the events or stimuli used in those studies were not sufficiently emotional to resemble real life. That poses a dilemma for researchers: On the one hand, field studies looking at memory for real life emotional events lack rigorous experimental control in general and a baseline in particular (i.e., it is difficult to know what really happened). On the other hand, for obvious ethical reasons one cannot manipulate memory for really traumatic events in the laboratory. The two studies of memory errors in the present issue have partly solved this dilemma by relying on memories for highly significant and shocking news events. The advantage is that it is relatively certain from media reports what really happened, while studies on flashbulb memories (Wright & Gaskell, 1995) indicate that hearing these events for the first time leads to reports of high emotionality (e.g., Conway et al., 1994).

In their contribution, Levine and Bluck looked at memories for hearing the verdict in the O. J. Simpson trial—an event viewed as significant by many North Americans. The authors' goal was to test the idea that valence matters for the extent to which reconstructive activities in memory lead to errors. They cleverly made use of the fact that hearing the outcome of the O. J. Simpson case led to different emotions in different people: some felt negative (sadness/anger), but others felt positive (happiness) about the verdict. Levine and Bluck's results show that positive people were more prone to making memory errors after 2 and 14 months than negative people. Apparently, happy people relied on a more schematic mode of information processing than people in a negative mood.

Levine and Bluck looked at naturally occurring memory errors, that is, they did nothing to suggest false information other than including foils in a recognition task. In contrast, Nourkova, Bernstein, and Loftus employed a much stronger manipulation. First, they asked their Russian participants to describe their memories of either the bombings of an apartment complex in Moscow or the planes crashing in the World Trade Center towers in New York. Six months later, the authors suggested to their participants that they had described a wounded animal in their first report. One eighth of the participants that recalled the Moscow bombings accepted this suggestion and subsequently described details of the false animal memory, whereas none of the participants in the WTC group did. Nourkova et al. acknowledge that 12.5% is not a very large proportion. Their point is, however, that misinformation even works when memories are about real life, highly emotional events.

Implications

More than a decade has passed since the debate about repression and malleability of traumatic memory reached its heated peak. The studies in the present special issue clearly show that the field has moved from establishing that both forgetting and falsely remembering emotional events is possible to attempting to pinpoint the mechanisms underlying these phenomena. Still, it is equally clear that many questions remain, and more research is needed to answer them.

As for forgetting, both Barnier, Hung, and Conway's work on retrieval-induced forgetting (RIF) and McNally et al.'s study on directed forgetting (DF) show that these paradigms can be successfully applied to emotional material. Barnier, Hung, and Conway are the first to report RIF in autobiographical memory. Their findings indicate that the highly complex and self-referential nature of autobiographical memories does not provide a boundary condition for obtaining an effect, as has sometimes been suggested (e.g., Macrae & Roseveare, 2002). McNally et al.'s finding that participants reporting repressed or recovered memories do not seem to possess special forgetting skills stresses the importance of investigating alternative explanations for why some people recover memories of abuse. The results of both studies are exiting and will spur on others in this area. In particular, researchers will want to know what mechanisms are responsible for the effects. Although the studies built upon work using techniques suggestive of an explanation in terms of (retrieval) inhibition (e.g., Anderson & Spellman, 1995), this does not necessarily mean that such a mechanism can be inferred from all results obtained with forgetting paradigms. We will not reiterate the excellent discussion of this topic offered by Barnier, Hung and Conway, but wish to stress that unless alternative explanations can be dismissed, researchers should remain cautious (see MacLeod, Dodd, Sheard, Wilson & Bibi, 2003, for a critical discussion of the concept of inhibition).

The three studies on repressive coping in this issue show that repressors are better at directed forgetting, but only for self-referent information under private conditions (Myers & Derakshan); that they are skilled at suppressing an unwanted negative, but not positive autobiographical memory (Barnier, Levin, & Maher) and that their unwillingness to process negative feedback at retrieval plays a role in their relatively poor recall of negative words (Shane & Peterson). These studies help to build a cognitive profile of what it is like to be a repressor. Repressive coping style is associated with poor health outcomes (Myers, 2000) so it is interesting to see how the results of these studies can help account for this association. If repressors truly experience less frequent intrusions of unwanted memories in consciousness, then they may be less prone to developing disorders that are characterised by frequent unwanted memories, such as posttraumatic stress disorder.

The studies of Levine and Bluck and Nourkova et al. confirm that emotional memory is malleable. Levine and Bluck's finding that positive rather than negative event valence gave rise to more errors in memory is interesting. Their interpretation that being in a positive or negative mood renders different styles of information processing calls for systematic research into how different discrete emotions affect memory. Finally, the critical aspect of Nourkova et al.'s study is that it was about very emotional memories. This study adds to a growing body of research showing that false information (details or entire memories) may be incorporated in autobiographical memory, and that emotion does not protect against it.

All in all, the studies in the present Special Issue show how emotional events may be forgotten and misremembered. Both the methods employed and the results obtained provide an excellent starting point for further unravelling the mechanisms underlying omissions and distortions in emotional memory. We expect that researchers will follow this lead and continue to pursue the important question of what causes emotional memory failures.

REFERENCES

Anderson, M. C., Bjork, R. A., & Bjork, E. L. (1994). Remembering can cause forgetting: Retrieval dynamics in long-term memory. *Journal of Experimental Psychology: Learning, Memory, and Cognition*, *20*, 1063–1087.

Anderson, M. C., & Spellman, B. A. (1995). On the status of inhibitory mechanisms in cognition: Memory retrieval as a model case. *Psychological Review*, *102*, 68–100.

Cloitre, M. (1998). Intentional forgetting and clinical disorders. In J. M. Golding (Ed.), *Intentional forgetting: Interdisciplinary approaches* (pp. 395–412). Mahwah, NJ: Erlbaum.

Conway, M. A., Anderson, S. J., Larsen, S. F., Donnely, C. M., McDaniel, M. A., McClelland, A. G. R., Rawles, R. E., & Logie, R. H. (1994). The formation of flashbulb memories. *Memory and Cognition*, *22*, 326–343.

Levy, B. J., & Anderson, M. C. (2002). Inhibitory processes and the control of memory retrieval. *Trends in Cognitive Sciences*, *6*, 299–305.

Loftus, E. F. (1997). Creating childhood memories. *Applied Cognitive Psychology* [Special Issue], *11*, S75–S86.

MacLeod, C. M., Dodd, M. D., Wilson, D. E., & Bibi, U. (2003). In opposition to inhibition. In B. H. Ross (Ed.), *The psychology of learning and motivation* (Vol. 43, pp. 163–214). San Diego, CA: Academic Press.

Macrae, C. N., & Roseveare, T. A. (2002). I was always on my mind: The self and temporary forgetting. *Psychonomic Bulletin and Review*, *9*, 611–614.

McNally, R. J. (2003). *Remembering trauma*. Cambridge, MA: Belknap Press/Harvard University Press.

Myers, L. B. (2000). Identifying repressors: A methodological issue for health psychology. *Psychology and Health*, *15*, 205–214.

Myers, L. B., Brewin, C. R., & Power, M. J. (1998). Repressive coping and the directed forgetting of emotional material. *Journal of Abnormal Psychology*, *107*, 141–148.

Ross, C. A. (2001). *Bluebird: Deliberate creation of multiple personality by psychiatrists* Richardson, TX: Manitou Communications

Wegner, D. M. (1989). *White bears and other unwanted thoughts: Suppression, obsession, and the psychology of mental control*. New York: Penguin.

Wright, D. B., & Gaskell, G. D. (1995). Flashbulb memories: Conceptual and methodological issues. *Memory*, *3*, 67–80.

Zur, J. N. (1998). *Violent memories: Mayan war widows in Guatemala*. Oxford, UK: Westview Press.

COGNITION AND EMOTION, 2004, *18* (4), 457–477

Retrieval-induced forgetting of emotional and unemotional autobiographical memories

Amanda J. Barnier and Lynette Hung
University of New South Wales, Sydney, Australia

Martin A. Conway
University of Durham, UK

This experiment extended the retrieval-induced forgetting (RIF) procedure from simple, episodic information to emotional and unemotional autobiographical memories. In the elicitation phase, participants generated specific memories from their past in response to negative, neutral, or positive category cues. In the retrieval-practice phase, they practised retrieving (and elaborated further on) some of the memories for some of the categories. In the final test phase, they tried to recall all memories. Memories that received retrieval practice were recalled more often on final test than baseline memories, whereas memories that were not practised, yet competed with practised memories via a shared category cue, were recalled less often than baseline memories. We discuss the roles of inhibition, competition, emotion, and self-relevance, and consider what laboratory manipulations of memory might reveal about everyday and pathological personal memory.

In recent years, researchers of human memory have recognised that forgetting some events from the past may be just as important as remembering others. Forgetting acts in part as an updating mechanism to reduce the impact of past, irrelevant experience on current, relevant activity (Bjork, 1989). Forgetting may serve also as a coping mechanism, which allows individuals to avoid memories that are threatening or disruptive to the self (Christianson & Engelberg, 1996; Erdelyi, 1990). In other words, rather than representing a cognitive failure, the ability to forget memories from the past may be crucial to explicit or implicit personal goals. This view is consistent with clinical reports that individuals with

---

Correspondence should be addressed to Amanda J. Barnier, School of Psychology, University of New South Wales, Sydney, NSW 2052, Australia; e-mail: A.Barnier@unsw.edu.au

This research is part of a larger project by Amanda Barnier and Martin Conway into the nature of autobiographical remembering and it was supported by an Australian Research Council Queen Elizabeth II Fellowship and Large Grant to Amanda Barnier and a Social and Economic Research Council of the United Kingdom Grant (No. R000239395) to Martin Conway. We are grateful for that support. We are grateful also to Rochelle Cox and Lyndel Mayoh for research assistance.

http://www.tandf.co.uk/journals/pp/02699931.html DOI:10.1080/02699930341000392

posttraumatic stress disorder may deliberately and persistently suppress thoughts and memories of their trauma, that individuals with functional amnesia and dissociative identity disorder appear wholly unaware of large parts of their autobiographical history, and that victims of childhood abuse suddenly and unexpectedly remember previously unrecalled experiences that they believe occurred years, if not decades, earlier (for reviews, see Brewin, 2001; Kihlstrom & Schacter, 1995; Koutstaal & Schacter, 1997; Wenzlaff & Wegner, 2000). Although such extreme forgetting is relatively rare and alternative explanations have been suggested (e.g., McNally, 2003; Pope, Hudson, Bodkin, & Olivia, 1998; Spanos, 1996), these phenomena raise important questions about the control that people have over what they remember and forget from their past.

The notion that individuals intentionally forget potentially disruptive thoughts and experiences is consistent with Freud's original definition of repression as ''turning something away, and keeping it at a distance from the conscious'' (Freud, 1915/1957, p. 147; see also Bowers & Farvolden, 1996; Conway, 2001a; Erdelyi, 1990; but see Holmes, 1990). It is consistent also with models of autobiographical memory that highlight motivational influences on personal remembering (e.g., Conway, 2001b; Conway & Pleydell-Pearce, 2000; McAdams, 2001; Singer & Salovey, 1993). For instance, Conway and Pleydell-Pearce (2000) proposed that autobiographical remembering occurs within a self-memory system (SMS), which includes the *working self* and an *autobiographical knowledge base*. The working self encompasses (among other things) a complex hierarchy of activated personal goals. The autobiographical knowledge base contains knowledge that is organised in terms of specificity (viz., lifetime periods, general events, sensory-perceptual episodic memory) and linked together into knowledge structures. Specific personal memories are conceptualised as stable patterns of activation across the knowledge base, which are created when the working self probes the knowledge base with successively elaborate cues until a pattern of activation is formed that satisfies working self goals. Memories can be generated also in response to highly specific cues, as long as the activated knowledge becomes linked to working self goals. In other words, executive processes that control memory generation are inextricably linked with current goals of the self. Also, importantly, these processes can inhibit (as well as facilitate), such that knowledge that is discrepant with or threatens the self may be actively prevented from reaching consciousness.

Within such models, autobiographical forgetting is conceptualised as goal-directed, although not necessarily within conscious control (Barnier, Conway, Mayoh, Speyer, & Avizmil, 2004; Erdelyi, 2001) and as recruiting inhibitory mechanisms that give rise to normal, and potentially abnormal, patterns of forgetting. Goal-directed forgetting via inhibitory processing has been explored using experimental procedures that attempt to create forgetting in the laboratory. For instance, in directed forgetting, participants are asked to recall stimuli they have been instructed to forget or remember (e.g., Barnier et al., 2004; Conway,

Harries, Noyes, Racsma'ny, & Frankish, 2000; MacLeod, 1998). In post-hypnotic amnesia, participants receive a suggestion that following hypnosis they will be unable to remember some, but not other, information or events (e.g., Barnier, 2002a; Cox & Barnier, 2003; Kihlstrom, 1980, 1985). And in retrieval-induced forgetting, participants repeatedly retrieve some information or events at the expense of other, related material (e.g., Anderson, Bjork, & Bjork, 1994; Anderson & Spellman, 1995; Perfect, Moulin, Conway, & Perry, 2002).

The selective impairment of ''to-be-forgotten'' (relative to ''to-be-remembered'') information created by these procedures has been conceptualised as ''inhibition''. But inhibition is interpreted in at least two ways and rests on a distinction between the potential availability of material in memory and its current accessibility (Tulving & Pearlstone, 1966). Memories that are available and accessible can be consciously brought to awareness (as indexed by explicit memory tests); memories that are available but not currently accessible remain outside of awareness but may influence ongoing experience (as indexed by implicit memory tests; Schacter, 1987); and memories that are neither available nor accessible influence neither conscious nor unconscious processing. Thus, inhibition is seen as either reducing the accessibility, but not availability, of information for retrieval (''retrieval inhibition''; MacLeod, 1998), or as reducing or deactivating the availability of the representation itself. The distinction between accessibility and availability is important because it highlights whether the ''forgotten'' information is only temporarily inaccessible to conscious recall or more permanently impaired (Bjork & Bjork, 1996; Kihlstrom & Barnhardt, 1993; Tulving & Pearlstone, 1966). This distinction has been highlighted also in discussions of clinical disorders of autobiographical memory and cases of ''repressed memory'' (Christianson & Engelberg, 1996; Kihlstrom & Schacter, 1995). Reductions in availability entail the strongest, mechanistic, and perhaps most unambiguous, form of inhibition.

Retrieval-induced forgetting (RIF) is one experimental procedure that reliably produces forgetting and, according to Anderson and his colleagues, operates at the level of availability (Anderson, Bjork, & Bjork, 2000; Anderson et al., 1994; Anderson & Spellman, 1995). In this procedure, participants initially study a series of category cue-exemplar word pairs (e.g., fruit-orange, fruit-apple). During the critical phase, participants perform repeated directed retrieval-practice on half of the exemplars from half of the categories via category-stem cued recall (e.g., fruit-or____). Finally, participants are re-presented with the entire list of category cue words and asked to recall all of the exemplars associated with each category cue. The impact of practising some words is measured against a baseline of words that are unpractised but related to practised words via a shared category cue, as well as words that are unpractised and unrelated to practised words (related to a different category cue). Using this procedure, Anderson et al. (1994, Experiment 1) reported that whereas participants' final recall of practised words (65–80%) was higher (i.e., facilitated) than their recall of unpractised unrelated words (40–50%), their recall of unpractised related words (30–40%) was lower (i.e., inhibited). RIF's deactivation of the representations themselves is demonstrated by later findings that final recall remains impaired even when tested with a novel, independent cue (the "independent probe technique"; Anderson & Spellman, 1995; but see Perfect et al., 2002). Thus, RIF appears to be the paradoxical (and seemingly unintentional, unconscious, and effortless) result of attempts to remember. Competition, rather than an explicit intention to forget, is the crucial factor that deactivates memory representations. Unpractised, yet competing, memories interfere with practised and wanted memories, and are inhibited to prevent recall of the unwanted memories (Anderson et al., 1994; Anderson & Spellman, 1995). Indeed, forgetting is maximised when exemplars are strongly associated to the common category cue, and abolished when exemplars are weakly associated or can be integrated (Anderson & McCulloch, 1999).

There is a strong view that experimental memory procedures, such as RIF, may reveal how and why individuals forget autobiographical events. For instance, Moulin et al. (2002) described RIF as a "paradigm that is ideal for assessing inhibition in episodic memory" (p. 863), and Anderson (2001) argued that the inhibitory processing indexed by RIF "may form the basis of some instances of traumatic forgetting" (p. 185; see also Anderson & Levy, 2002; Barnier, 2002b; Barnier & McConkey, 1999; Bjork, Bjork, & Anderson, 1998; Conway, 2001a; Koutstaal & Schacter, 1997; but see Kihlstrom, 2002). This claim remains untested, since most research has focused on only relatively simple, nonpersonal, and emotionally neutral information (e.g., word lists). Autobiographical memories, in contrast, are complex, self-generated, personally relevant, and emotionally significant to the individual. These differences may limit the degree to which the processes that operate successfully on simple material will influence personal memories. Emotionality (emotional vs. unemotional) and emotional valence (negative vs. neutral vs. positive) of targeted memories are particularly relevant since: (1) negative experiences are assumed to be upsetting or threatening to the self and individuals strive to forget them (for a discussion of the role of individual differences in forgetting, see Davis, 1990; Weinberger, 1990); and (2) traumatic events are well remembered in some circumstances but completely or partially forgotten in others (compared with neutral events; for a review, see Christianson, 1992; Christianson & Engelberg, 1999).

A handful of studies has extended RIF beyond word lists, but its impact on more complex, socially relevant, and emotional material is mixed. Macrae and MacLeod (1999) adapted RIF to an impression formation task in which practised and unpractised items were traits that characterised two men, and to a mock geography exam in which practised and unpractised items were facts about two fictitious tropical items. They reported reliable RIF for both tasks and both sets of material. MacLeod (2002) examined RIF in eyewitness memory, and reported that individuals' ability to recall some items stolen in a (simulated) burglary and some features of the suspects was impaired by repeated retrieval of other items and other features (see also Bylin & Christianson, 2002; Shaw, Bjork, & Handal, 1995). In contrast, Macrae and Roseveare (2002) examined RIF for two sets of gift items following an encoding manipulation; during the learning phase participants were instructed to imagine either that they themselves, a best friend, or an unspecified other had purchased the gifts. Macrae and Roseveare (2002) reported standard RIF in the best friend and other conditions, but not in the self-referent condition. They argued that self-relevant material might be protected from temporary forgetting via distinctive processing during encoding. Finally, Amir, Coles, Brigidi, and Foa (2001) tested individuals with social phobia and nonanxious controls using negative social words, positive social words, and nonsocial words as practised and unpractised items. Nonanxious controls demonstrated RIF for negative, positive, and nonsocial words. Social phobics, however, only showed RIF for positive and nonsocial words; practice did not inhibit recall of unpractised negative social words. Research within a related laboratory paradigm, directed forgetting (DF), has suggested a similar asymmetry across emotional and unemotional material. Across six experiments, Barnier et al. (2004) extended DF to autobiographical memories. Participants were asked to recall specific negative, positive, and neutral personal memories from their past in response to 15 cue words (list 1). They then received a DF instruction: Half were told to forget these memories and half were told to remember them. Both groups then recalled a second set of memories to 15 new cue words (list 2). On a final free recall test, participants given forget instructions typically recalled fewer list 1 memories than participants given remember instructions. Importantly, across all six experiments Barnier et al. (2004) failed to generate DF of negative (as opposed to neutral and positive) memories (for directed forgetting of emotional words, see Myers, Brewin, & Power, 1998; Power, Dalgleish, Claudio, & Tata, & Kentish, 2000).

This experiment extended Anderson et al.'s (1994) RIF procedure to emotional and unemotional autobiographical memories. Participants recalled 30 specific autobiographical memories from their past in response to negative, neutral, and positive category cue words. They learned the associations between the category cue words and their autobiographical memories, and then practised retrieving some, but not other, memories. In the retrieval-practice task, participants repeatedly attempted to recall half of their associated memories for half of the categories. Recall of these memories was cued three times, and each time participants were asked to provide additional information about the event. A final recall test indexed participants' recall of practised memories from practised categories (Rp+), unpractised memories from practised categories (Rp−), and unpractised memories from unpractised categories (Nrp). Based on findings with word pair and more complex stimuli, we expected that autobiographical forgetting (as indexed by final recall) would be influenced by repeated retrieval practice. We expected that Rp+ memories would be facilitated (higher final recall) relative to Nrp memories, but that Rp− memories would be impaired (lower final recall) relative to Nrp (and Rp+) memories, because they compete at retrieval with Rp+ memories via their shared category cue. Based on Barnier et al.'s (2004) finding that negative memories are less susceptible to directed forgetting (a procedure which also involves competition between wanted and unwanted material), we expected that retrieval practice in RIF might influence neutral and positive memories more so than negative memories.

METHOD

Participants and design

A total of 40 (10 male, 30 female) undergraduate psychology students from the University of New South Wales, Sydney, Australia were tested in a (3) (memory response: Rp+ vs. Rp− vs. Nrp) × (3) (emotional valence: negative vs. neutral vs. positive) within-subjects design. They participated in return for credit towards their psychology course, and ranged in age from 17 to 24 years (M = 19.30, SD = 1.91).

Materials and apparatus

Nine category cue words were used to elicit memories. They were chosen because in previous research (Barnier et al., 2004) they were rated as reliably negative, neutral, or positive, and elicited specific and reliably negative, neutral, or positive memories from the majority of participants. The words were: (negative) horrified, sickness, tragedy; (neutral) hardworking, patient, polite; (positive), entertaining, excitement, happy. The nine words were divided into three sets of three words each (one each negative, neutral, positive), and combined into three counterbalancing orders in which each word set acted as Rp, Nrp, and filler category cue words (see Appendix). Participants were randomly assigned to one of three word order counterbalancing conditions.[1]

The experimenter verbally presented the category cue words. Unless otherwise stated, the cue words were presented one at a time in random order, with the constraints that filler words appeared randomly at the beginning and end of each phase, and the same cue word never appeared twice in a row. Participants' verbal responses during elicitation and final test were recorded using a Sony audiocassette recorder. Response latencies during elicitation, learning, retrieval-practice, and final test were timed using a stopwatch.

[1] Initial analyses of the major variables indicated that word order counterbalancing condition did not influence participants' performance, and will not be considered further.

Procedure

The experiment involved five phases: (1) elicitation; (2) learning; (3) retrieval-practice; (4) final test; and (5) postexperimental inquiry. The procedure was based as closely as possible on Anderson et al.'s (1994) methodology, with modifications only for the use of autobiographical memories as the target stimuli. Participants were tested in individual sessions with the experimenter, and sat facing the experimenter.

Elicitation. To begin, participants were told that they were taking part in an experiment examining individual differences in the ability to remember and think about autobiographical events. The experimenter said that she would verbally present cue words one at a time and their task was to generate specific memories from any part of their life in response to these words as quickly as possible. A specific memory was defined as ''a unique, single event that you have experienced, typically measured in seconds, minutes, or even hours, but not days''. Participants were told also that the category cue words would be repeatedly presented and that they should generate different, unique memories to each presentation of the same cue word (as well as across different cue words). Participants were instructed to indicate when they had a specific, relevant memory in mind by saying ''yes''. To ensure that participants generated the required memories, participants were given as long as necessary to elicit each memory. Memory generation latency was measured from the offset of verbal category cue word presentation until participants said ''yes''. If participants said ''yes'', they gave a 10–15 word verbal description of their memory to the experimenter, estimated how old they were when the event occurred, and rated the memory in terms of clarity (''how clear is your memory of the event''; 1 = not at all clear, 7 = extremely clear) and emotional valence (''how positive or negative is your memory of this event''; 1 = very negative, 4 = neither negative nor positive, 7 = very positive). In addition, participants were asked to provide a ''personal word'' for each memory that would remind them of the event if asked about it again. Participants engaged in this cycle of generating, describing, dating, and rating memories until they had elicited a total of 30 memories to the nine category cues; four memories to each of three Rp category cue words (1 each negative, neutral, positive), four memories to each of three Nrp category cue words (1 each negative, neutral, positive), and two memories to each of three filler category cue words (1 each negative, neutral, positive).

Learning. In the next phase, participants learned the category cue word, personal word, and autobiographical memory associations so they could provide the correct memory when presented with the category cue words and personal words alone. In each learning trial, the experimenter verbally presented one of the category cue word-personal word-autobiographical memory associations (e.g., ''hardworking''-''exams''-''studying for my final exams'') and then paused for 20 seconds. Participants were instructed to use the 20 s to form a connection between the category cue word, their personal word, and their memory. The presentation order of the associations was block randomised to minimise connections between memories elicited from the same category cue word. Each block comprised one association from each Rp and Nrp category cue word, resulting in four blocks of six category cue word-personal word-autobiographical memory associations. Order of the associations within each block was random, with the constraints that throughout the learning list no two category cue words appeared consecutively more than twice and three filler associations (1 each negative, neutral, positive) appeared at the beginning and end of the learning list (see Appendix).

Retrieval-practice. Prior to the critical retrieval-practice phase, the experimenter randomly assigned participants to one of two retrieval practice orders (viz., practised 1st & 3rd memories or 2nd and 4th memories from each Rp category cue word).[2] The experimenter explained that in the next phase she would repeatedly present a number of the category cue word-personal word pairings, and their task was to respond to each presentation with the correct autobiographical memory. She said she would give them 20 s to try to retrieve the appropriate memory (rather than any alternative or new memory that fit the pairing). Retrieval-practice involved 36 trials and focused on two (out of four) memories associated with each of the three Rp category cue words (Rp+ memories), and the two memories associated with each of the three filler category cue words. The experimenter presented each category cue word-personal word pairing three times. Rp+ memories were practised in an expanding schedule separated by intervals in which other memories received practice. The first and second retrievals of each Rp+ memory occurred with an average of 6.50 intervening memories; the second and third retrievals occurred with an average of 11.83 intervening memories. In general, no two memories associated with the same category cue word were practised adjacently and the same sequences of retrieval practice trials were prevented from appearing consecutively by inserting filler memory trials. The first and last three trials were tests of randomly ordered filler memories (1 each negative, neutral, positive).

Participants were instructed to indicate when they recalled the correct associated memory by saying ''yes''. For all retrieval-practice trials, if participants said ''yes'', they were asked to report the memory. On the second practice trial, the experimenter asked participants to recall additional details about the event (''Are there any additional details you can remember about the event that you

[2] Initial analyses of the major variables indicated that retrieval-practice order did not influence participants' performance, and will not be considered further.

didn't recall before?'') On the third practice trial, the experimenter administered three standard probes for additional information irrespective of previous descriptions; these focused on physical surroundings (''Thinking about the event, tell me more about where you were, your physical surroundings''), interpersonal aspects (''Tell me more about the people you were with''), and emotional experiences (''Tell me more about how you felt''). If participants correctly reported their associated memory, the experimenter presented the next category cue word-personal word pairing. If participants failed to respond or reported an incorrect memory, she gave no specific feedback and presented the next pairing without asking the additional questions. At the conclusion of retrieval-practice, participants completed the two 5 min unrelated distraction tasks (number and name checking, ACER; L-shaped puzzle, Snodgrass & Burns, 1978).

Final test. Participants were re-presented with all nine category cue words and asked to recall all the memories associated with each word (max. 4 memories each for Rp and Nrp category cue words, max. 2 memories each for filler category cue words). Participants were given 60 s to recall all the memories they generated for each category cue word; they were not told the number of memories expected for each category. Participants verbally recalled memories without interruption until 60 s had elapsed. The experimenter then presented the next category cue word until the nine words had been presented.

Postexperimental enquiry. Participants were asked about their experiences during retrieval practice and final test. Specifically, they were asked how easy or difficult they found recalling some of the memories during retrieval-practice (1 = *extremely difficult*, 7 = *very easy*), how easy or difficult they found recalling their memories at the end of the experiment (1 = *extremely difficult*, 7 = *very easy*), and whether they found some memories easier to recall than others. Finally, participants were invited to ask questions, debriefed, and thanked for their participation.

RESULTS

Memories at elicitation

All participants generated the maximum of 30 memories to the category cue words: four memories to each of the three negative, neutral, and positive Rp category cue words, four memories to each of the three negative, neutral, and positive Nrp category cue words, and two memories to each of the negative, neutral, and positive filler category cue words. A (3) (memory response) × (3) (emotional valence) repeated-measures ANOVA of mean generation latency for these memories yielded only a significant main effect of emotional valence,

$F(2, 78) = 8.05$, $p = .001$, $\eta_p^2 = .171$.[3] No other main or interaction effects were significant. Participants took slightly longer to generate memories to neutral ($M = 16.54$, $SD = 8.07$) than to negative ($M = 13.45$, $SD = 7.15$) or positive ($M = 11.99$, $SD = 5.87$) category cue words, $t(39) = 3.14$, $p = .003$ and $t(39) = 4.08$, $p < .001$, respectively; this finding may reflect the extremely mild (and perhaps personally unimportant) nature of the neutral memories. Overall, participants generated the required number of memories within 10–15 s each.

Participants estimated the mean age of elicited memories (i.e., age at time of the event) and rated the clarity (1 = *not at all clear*, 7 = *very clear*) and valence (1 = *very negative*, 4 = *neither negative nor positive*, 7 = *very positive*) of their memories. Separate (3) (memory response) × (3) (emotional valence) repeated measures ANOVAs of these data yielded main effects of emotional valence for age of memories, clarity ratings, and valence ratings, $F(2, 78) = 7.37$, $p = .001$, $\eta^2 = .159$, $F(2, 78) = 5.83$, $p = .004$, $\eta^2 = .130$, and $F(2, 78) = 302.90$, $p < .001$, $\eta_p^2 = .886$, respectively. Participants generated slightly older memories to negative cue words ($M = 16.64$, $SD = 1.79$) than to neutral cue words ($M = 17.78$, $SD = 1.87$) and to positive cue words ($M = 17.37$, $SD = 2.22$), $t(39) = 4.83$, $p < .001$ and $t(39) = 2.43$, $p = .020$, respectively. Memories to positive cue words were a similar age to memories to neutral cue words, $t(39) = 1.66$, $p = .105$. They rated their memories to positive cue words ($M = 5.74$, $SD = 0.76$) as somewhat clearer than their memories to negative ($M = 5.43$, $SD = 0.81$) and neutral ($M = 5.45$, $SD = 0.76$) cue words, $t(39) = 2.98$, $p = .005$ and $t(39) = 2.84$, $p = .007$, respectively; they rated memories to neutral and negative cue words similarly, $t(39) = 0.13$, $p = .900$. Finally, participants rated their memories to negative cue words ($M = 2.56$, $SD = 0.64$) as more negative/less positive than their memories to neutral ($M = 3.94$, $SD = 0.63$) or positive ($M = 5.85$, $SD = 0.56$) cue words, $t(39) = 12.35$, $p < .001$ and $t(39) = 22.81$, $p < .001$, respectively. They in turn rated their memories to neutral cue words as more negative/less positive than their memories to positive cue words, $t(39) = 15.50$, $p < .001$. Overall, participants' memories were of a similar age (negative memories were slightly older) and generally very clear (positive memories were clearest). Also, negative, neutral, and positive category cue words elicited negative, neutral, and positive memories as intended.

Manipulation checks: Retrieval-practice performance

During retrieval-practice, participants recalled their associated (Rp+) memories when presented with category cue word-personal word pairings. Half the participants practised memories 1 and 3 from the practised category cue words and

[3] Partial eta squared (η_p^2) was used to estimate the strength of association for each effect in ANOVA. Tabachnick and Fidell (1996) recommended its use because, unlike eta squared (η^2), it is not influenced by the number and significance of other independent variables in the design.

half practised memories 2 and 4. A (3) (emotional valence) × 2 (practice order) repeated-measures ANOVA of participants' retrieval-practice success (operationalised as the percentage of trials on which they correctly recalled the appropriate Rp+ memory) yielded no significant main or interaction effects. Participants correctly recalled over 90% of Rp+ memories (*M* per cent = 94.72, *SD* = 12.32). As well as recalling the correct memories, on second practice trials participants provided additional information about the remembered event for 85% of Rp+ memories, and on third practice trials, they responded to probes about physical surroundings, interpersonal aspects, and emotional experiences for 68%, 50%, and 84% of Rp+ memories, respectively. Participants' ratings of the ease of recalling memories during the retrieval-practice phase ranged from 3 to 7 (1 = *extremely difficult*, 7 = *very easy*) and averaged 4.46 (*SD* = 1.10). Overall, during this phase, participants not only successfully retrieved their negative, neutral, and positive Rp+ memories, but also elaborated on them.

Final test

During final test, participants attempted to recall all of their associated memories to all (Rp, Nrp, and filler) category cue words. Memories were scored as correct if the memory description at final test corresponded to the memory description at elicitation. Although exact correspondences were not required, there had to be a clear relationship between the two (viz., they had to report at least some of the same information, and unambiguously refer to the same event). Table 1 presents the mean percentage of memories correctly recalled. Anderson et al.'s (1994) analyses of final recall included participants whose retrieval-practice success was greater than 80%. Thirty-six of our 40 participants exceeded this criterion and were included in the following analyses. A (3) (memory response) × (3) (emotional valence) within-subjects ANOVA of this data yielded significant main effects of memory response and emotional valence, $F(2, 70) = 28.96$, $p < .001$, $\eta_p^2 = .453$ and $F(2, 70) = 16.15$, $p < .001$, $\eta_p^2 = .316$, respectively; the interaction between memory response and emotional valence was not significant. Planned *t*-tests confirmed that participants recalled more Rp+ than Nrp memories, $t(35) = 4.98$, $p < .001$. However, they recalled fewer Rp− than Nrp memories, $t(35) = 4.12$, $p < .001$ (see Table 1). In other words, whereas memories practised during the retrieval-practice phase were facilitated on final test relative to the baseline of Nrp memories, memories that were unpractised, yet related to practised memories via a shared category cue, were impaired on final test relative to Nrp memories.

Focusing next on the impact of emotional valence, overall participants recalled fewer positive (*M* per cent = 65.63, *SD* = 18.99) than neutral (*M* per cent = 85.76, *SD* = 11.63) or negative (*M* percent = 76.74, *SD* = 14.38) memories, $t(35) = 5.70$, $p < .001$ and $t(35) = 2.79$, $p = .008$, respectively. They also recalled fewer negative than neutral memories, $t(35) = 2.92$, $p = .006$. In other words,

TABLE 1
Mean percentage (and standard deviations) of memories correctly recalled

Memory response	Overall	Emotional valence		
		Negative	*Neutral*	*Positive*
Rp+	88.89 (12.60)	84.72 (28.83)	97.22 (11.62)	84.72 (26.24)
Rp−	62.50 (20.07)	63.89 (32.97)	77.78 (27.89)	45.83 (38.50)
Nrp	75.93 (10.69)	79.17 (18.42)	82.64 (17.75)	65.97 (24.75)
Filler	92.13 (10.90)	94.44 (15.94)	100.00 (0.00)	81.94 (29.65)

Note: Rp+ = practised memories from practised category cue words; Rp− = unpractised memories from practised category cue words; Nrp = unpractised memories from unpractised category cue words. Consistent with Anderson et al. (1994), filler memories were excluded from the analyses.

participants were more likely to forget emotional (positive and negative) memories than unemotional (neutral) memories.

We also considered whether memory elaboration or output order could account for performance on final recall. During retrieval-practice, participants were asked to provide additional details about each event on the second practice trial, and to answer three standard probes about physical surroundings, interpersonal aspects, and emotional experiences on the third practice trial. A series of Pearson correlations between final test recall variables (Rp+, Rp−, and Nrp memories) and retrieval-practice elaboration variables (correct retrieval on trial 1, additional information on trial 2, and spatial, interpersonal, and emotional information on trial 3) indicated no significant relationships; correlations ranged between −.11 and .29 and all were nonsignificant ($p < .05$). Thus, elaboration during retrieval-practice was not responsible for superior recall of Rp+ memories at final test.

To assess possible output order effects, we followed Macrae and Roseveare's (2002) procedure of classifying participants according to whether their recall sequences commenced with Rp+ or Rp− items (see also Conway et al., 2000). First, we calculated the average recall positions of Rp+ and Rp− memories. For each Rp category cue word, the first recalled memory was assigned a score of "1", the second a score of "2", the third a score of "3", and the fourth a score of "4". Lower position scores indicated that memories were recalled earlier. The average position scores for Rp+ and Rp− memories were 2.00 ($SD = 0.38$) and 2.45 ($SD = 0.70$), respectively. We then subtracted the average recall position of Rp+ items from the average recall position of Rp− items and sorted participants using a median split of the difference score. This produced an "early Rp+" group ($n = 18$) and an "early Rp−" group ($n = 18$). We repeated the overall ANOVA for final recall data with output group as a between-subject factor and repeated the planned *t*-tests for early Rp+ and early Rp− groups

TABLE 2
Mean percentage (and standard deviations) of memories correctly recalled according to output order

	Output group	
Memory response	*Rp+ early*	*Rp− early*
Rp+	87.04 (13.47)	90.74 (11.75)
Rp−	62.96 (17.67)	62.04 (22.73)
Nrp	74.54 (11.95)	77.31 (9.40)

Note: Rp+ = practised memories from practised category cue words; Rp− = unpractised memories from practised category cue words; Nrp = unpractised memories from unpractised category cue words.

separately (see Table 2). There were no significant main or interaction effects for output group in the overall ANOVA. On the *t*-tests, participants recalled more Rp+ than Nrp memories [early Rp+: $t(17) = 3.04$, $p = .007$; early Rp−: $t(17) = 4.06$, $p = .001$], but fewer Rp− than Nrp memories [early Rp+: $t(17) = 2.65$, $p = .017$; early Rp−: $t(17) = 3.11$, $p = .006$], irrespective of order of recall. These findings imply that our RIF effect was not due to output interference during the final recall test.

Participants' ratings of the ease of recalling memories during final test ranged from 2 to 6 (1 = *extremely difficult*, 7 = *very easy*) and averaged 4.17 (SD = 1.18). When asked to comment on their recall experience, 5 (14%) participants said that they found it easier to recall practised memories, 11 (31%) said they found it easier to recall specific (vs. general) memories, 6 (17%) said they found recent memories easier, 15 (42%) said they found emotional (both positive and negative) memories easier, and 12 (33%) said they found emotional memories harder to recall (note, some participants gave more than one reason). Overall, participants found recalling memories a moderately difficult task, which many attributed to the nature of memories, rather than the retrieval practice of some memories.

DISCUSSION

This experiment yielded a standard retrieval-induced forgetting effect for autobiographical memories. On the final recall test, participants showed facilitation of memories repeatedly retrieved during retrieval practice (Rp+ > Nrp). Also, they showed impairment of memories that were not practised, but related to practised memories via a shared category cue (Rp− < Nrp). According to the logic of the RIF procedure, retrieving some autobiographical memories may unintentionally, and almost inevitably, inhibit other memories related to the same retrieval cue. The degree of impairment of Rp− memories was noteworthy: 10–15% below the baseline of Nrp memories and 20–25% below practised Rp+ memories. This pattern is consistent with, and significantly extends, research involving simple (word list) and more complex material (Anderson et al., 1994, 2000; Anderson & Spellman, 1995; Bylin & Christianson, 2002; MacLeod, 2002; Macrae & MacLeod, 1999; Shaw et al., 1995).

Does this finding genuinely reflect inhibition? Anderson and colleagues argued that the classic RIF pattern of Rp− < Nrp is due to inhibition operating at the level of availability. They claimed that competition between wanted and unwanted material reduces the availability of unwanted, competing representations (Anderson et al., 1994, 2000; Anderson & Spellman, 1995). Output interference offers an alternative, noninhibitory explanation. Retrieval of Rp+ memories may interfere with other memories, not via inhibition, but by overshadowing recall of other category items. Our post-hoc analyses of output order (which used average recall positions and compared early Rp+ vs. early Rp− groups; see also Conway et al., 2000; Macrae & Roseveare, 2002) did not support this interpretation. Future extensions of RIF to autobiographical memory could formally manipulate output order on final test by providing both the category cue and an additional cue to either Rp+ or Rp- memories. For instance, the personal word we used during retrieval-practice could be used also on final recall to control output order and separate output interference from genuine inhibitory effects.

If RIF of autobiographical memories reflects inhibition, what exactly is inhibited? Anderson and Spellman (1995) argued that ‘‘if a representation is truly inhibited [at the availability level], performance impairments arising from that inhibition should generalise to any cue used to test that item’’ (p. 92; see also Perfect et al., 2002). In other words, if Rp− memories are impaired on all tests, then RIF inhibits availability. But if Rp− memories are impaired only in response to the original category cue, then RIF inhibits accessibility, not availability (as in list-method directed forgetting, Conway et al., 2000; MacLeod, 1998). Anderson and Spellman (1995) tested this with their independent probe technique, which indexes memories with novel cues that are semantically related to the target memories, but are not part of the original cue-memory pairings (e.g., if FOOD-STRAWBERRY is an original pairing, RED is used as the independent probe to cue STRAWBERRY on the final test). They reported Rp− < Nrp irrespective of the retrieval cue—original or novel—used to test memory. In a different approach, Perfect et al. (2002) tested whether RIF impairs performance on implicit memory tasks (as well as on the standard explicit recall task). If Rp− memories are impaired on explicit, but not implicit, tests, then again RIF inhibits accessibility, not availability (as in list-method directed forgetting; Basden, Basden, & Gargano, 1993). Interestingly, they reported Rp− < Nrp in standard cued recall and conceptual implicit memory (category generation, category matching), but not in perceptual implicit memory (stem completion, and perceptual identification).

We did not use independent cues or implicit tasks because it was not immediately obvious how to adapt them to complex autobiographical memories. The independent probe technique, for instance, uses items that can be cued via their original category (e.g., for STRAWBERRY, FOOD) and by a novel, semantically related category not previously encountered in the experiment (e.g., for STRAWBERRY, RED). A valid test of cue independence assumes that the target items are reasonably (and perhaps equally) accessible with the novel category cue. Thinking of the present experiment, participants generated autobiographical memories to cues, such as ''happy'', ''hardworking'', and ''tragedy''. Would semantically related cues such as ''pleased'', ''industrious'', and ''catastrophe'' work, and work for everyone, given that autobiographical memories are organised within a complex hierarchy of life period, temporal, thematic, emotional, and perceptual-sensory information (Conway, 2001b; Conway & Pleydell-Pearce, 2000)? For instance, a memory elicited to ''tragedy'' may be most strongly associated with (and thus most accessible via) a particular time period or life theme. Research on autobiographical event clusters, which asks participants to generate chains of memories to an initial cue and examines their emotional, thematic, and personal significance threads (Wright & Nunn, 2000), might assist a valid extension of the independent probe technique to autobiographical memories.

Implicit autobiographical memory tasks also need consideration since the notion itself is conceptually counterintuitive (Conway & Pleydell-Pearce, 2000) and standard measures developed for word stimuli are inappropriate. Barnier (2002a; see also Cox & Barnier, 2003) developed a social judgement task to measure the impact of posthypnotic amnesia on autobiographical memories, which drew on conceptually similar tasks in implicit social cognition (e.g., the false-fame effect; Jacoby, Kelley, Brown, & Jasechko, 1989; Squire & McKee, 1992). Following a standard free recall task, participants made an evaluative judgement (likelihood) about their own autobiographical events and foil events. Although participants' free recall of the events targeted by posthypnotic amnesia was impaired, information from the ''forgotten'' events influenced their likelihood ratings. Development of such implicit tasks may provide another means to evaluate the form of inhibition operating in RIF of autobiographical memories.

The impairment of related, but unpractised memories in RIF suggests that competition is an important, if not crucial, prerequisite for forgetting. Participants did not intend to forget Rp− memories. Rather, practising the Rp+ memories created the conditions that triggered inhibition of Rp− memories. Anderson et al. (1994) argued that inhibitory processes are activated and directed at unwanted, yet competing, memories to reduce their interference with wanted memories at retrieval. This prime role of competition is seen also in directed forgetting (Bjork et al., 1998). Notably, in both procedures, wanted (practised) and unwanted (unpractised) memories must be sufficiently related, but not completely related, to create competition and trigger inhibition. Competition, and thus inhibition, is reduced when memories can be integrated in some way (Barnier et al., 2004; Conway et al., 2000; see also Anderson & McCulloch, 1999).

Competition versus integration is particularly important to autobiographical RIF since personal memories are highly organised and related with the autobiographical knowledge base (Conway, 2001b; Conway & Pleydell-Pearce, 2000). Memories are related not only via sensory or emotional features, but also at the level of lifetime periods and general events. Organisation may protect memories from inhibition. For instance, Barnier et al. (2004) reported that directed forgetting was abolished when two sets of autobiographical memories were thematically related (for similar findings for words, see Conway et al., 2000). Participants who generated one set of "high school memories" and one set of "holiday memories" showed forgetting, whereas those who generated two sets of "high school memories" (which could be integrated into one lifetime period), did not. Alternatively, organisation may promote inhibition. For instance, Wright and Nunn (2000) reported that memories within autobiographical event clusters were more similar on dimensions of emotionality, personal significance, and clarity than they were to memories from other clusters. Thus, whole clusters of autobiographical memories may be easier to target for inhibition because they are naturally related and can be segregated from other clusters of memories.

We expected that the impact of retrieval practice would be moderated by emotional valence, with negative memories less likely forgotten than neutral and positive memories. Although retrieval practice impaired unpractised memories, emotional valence influenced recall irrespective of practice status. On the final test, participants recalled fewer positive than negative memories, and fewer negative than neutral memories. In other words, they recalled fewer emotional than unemotional memories. Although this effect, independent of practice, may reflect inherent differences in the accessibility, organisation, and personal significance of emotional and unemotional memories, it supports the view that emotional memories are retained and recalled differently to neutral memories (Christianson, 1992; Christianson & Engelberg, 1999). In particular, it suggests that individuals avoid retrieving emotional experiences. A similar emotional memory bias has been shown in people with a "repressive coping style" (Weinberger, 1990), who avoid thinking about or recalling negative childhood events, negative recent events, and negative, self-descriptive adjectives (Barnier, Levin, & Maher, this issue; Davis, 1990; Myers et al., 1998).

The finding that participants recalled fewer negative than neutral memories on the final test is inconsistent with experiments involving directed forgetting of positive, neutral, and negative autobiographical memories. Barnier et al. (2004) reported that negative memories were relatively immune to the forget instruction. This variability, both across and irrespective of memory manipulations, suggests that a sole focus on emotionality is too simplistic. Remembering and forgetting may be equally, if not more influenced by self-relevance; memories that are self-defining, self-relevant, or rehearsed as part of an individual's life story (McAdams, 2001) may be difficult to forget irrespective of valence (see also Conway & Pleydell-Pearce, 2000). At first glance this proposal is consistent with Macrae and Roseveare's (2002) finding of no RIF effect for self-relevant material. But then why did we find RIF for autobiographical memories since they are by definition self-relevant? We suggest two reasons. First, as Macrae and Roseveare (2002) acknowledged, their results probably reflect distinctive encoding operations rather than genuine differences in self-relevance. Second, any set of autobiographical memories will vary in their importance to the self and so too will the rate at which particular memories within the set are remembered or forgotten; memories that are central to working self goals may be inoculated from inhibition more so than memories that are relevant, but not crucial to the self (Conway, 2001b; Conway & Pleydell-Pearce, 2000; Weinberger, 1990). Future research should consider not only how RIF influences autobiographical memories, but why some memories are inhibited and not others.

The main finding of this experiment is that the RIF procedure impaired emotional and unemotional autobiographical memories. This suggests that the processes that operate successfully on simple material also influence personal memories. Since our results may be due to inhibition of availability or accessibility (or some other process), future research should seek the locus of forgetting, as well as its relationship to other forms of laboratory forgetting. Laying aside the precise mechanism, the conditions modelled by RIF might be one way that individuals shape their life story and manage unwanted memories. By rehearsing memories that support a positive rather than negative, ordered rather than disordered, life story, they may become highly accessible. Each time these memories are accessed they may reinforce the inhibition of competing, undesirable autobiographical knowledge. In this way, forgetting may be goal-directed, but unintentional. Whether or not this account is valid, extending RIF (and related procedures) to emotional autobiographical memories brings us one step closer to understanding everyday and pathological patterns of personal memory.

REFERENCES

Amir, N., Coles, M. E., Brigidi, B., & Foa, E. B. (2001). The effect of practice on recall of emotional information in individuals with generalized social phobia. *Journal of Abnormal Psychology, 110*, 76–82.

Anderson, M. C. (2001). Active forgetting: Evidence for functional inhibition as a source of memory failure. *Journal of Aggression, Maltreatment and Trauma, 4*, 185–210.

Anderson, M. C., Bjork, R. A., Bjork, E. L. (1994). Remembering can cause forgetting: Retrieval dynamics in long-term memory. *Journal of Experimental Psychology: Learning, Memory, and Cognition, 20*, 1063–1087.

Anderson, M. C., Bjork, E. L., & Bjork, R. A. (2000). Retrieval-induced forgetting: Evidence for a recall-specific mechanism. *Psychonomic Bulletin and Review*, *7*, 522–530.

Anderson, M. C., & Levy, B. (2002). Inhibitory processes and the control of memory retrieval. *Trends in Cognitive Science*, *6*, 299–305.

Anderson, M. C., & McCulloch, K. C. (1999). Integration as a general boundary condition on retrieval-induced forgetting. *Journal of Experimental Psychology: Learning, Memory, and Cognition*, *25*, 608–629.

Anderson, M. C., & Spellman, B. A. (1995). On the status of inhibitory mechanisms in cognition: Memory retrieval as a model case. *Psychological Review*, *102*, 68–100.

Barnier, A. J. (2002a). Posthypnotic amnesia for autobiographical episodes: A laboratory model of functional amnesia? *Psychological Science*, *13*, 232–237.

Barnier, A. J. (2002b). Remembering and forgetting autobiographical events: Instrumental uses of hypnosis. *Contemporary Hypnosis*, *19*, 51–61.

Barnier, A. J., Conway, M. A., Mayoh, L., Speyer, J., & Avizmil, O. (2004). *Directed forgetting of autobiographical memories*. Manuscript under review.

Barnier, A. J., Levin, K., & Maher, A. (this issue). Suppressing thoughts of past events: Are repressive copers good suppressors? *Cognition and Emotion*, *18*, 513–531.

Barnier, A. J., & McConkey, K. M. (1999). Autobiographical remembering and forgetting: What can hypnosis tell us? *International Journal of Clinical and Experimental Hypnosis*, *47*, 267–285.

Basden, B. H., Basden, D. R., & Gargano, G. J. (1993). Directed forgetting in implicit and explicit memory tests: A comparison of methods. *Journal of Experimental Psychology: Learning, Memory, and Cognition*, *19*, 603–616.

Bjork, R. A. (1989). Retrieval inhibition as an adaptive mechanism in human memory. In H. L. Roediger III & F. I. M. Craik (Eds.), *Varieties of memory and consciousness: Essays in honor of Endel Tulving* (pp. 309–330). Hillsdale, NJ: Erlbaum.

Bjork, E. L., & Bjork, R. A. (1996). Continuing influences of to-be-forgotten information. *Consciousness and Cognition*, *5*, 176–196.

Bjork, R. A., Bjork, E. L., & Anderson, M. C. (1998). Varieties of goal-directed forgetting. In J. M. Golding & C. M. MacLeod (Eds.), *Intentional forgetting: Interdisciplinary approaches* (pp. 103–137). Mahwah, NJ: Erlbaum.

Bowers, K. S., & Farvolden, P. (1996). Revisiting a century-old Freudian slip: From suggestion disavowed to the truth repressed. *Psychological Bulletin*, *119*, 355–380.

Brewin, C. R. (2001). Memory processes in posttraumatic stress disorder. *International Review of Psychiatry*, *13*, 159–163.

Bylin, S., & Christianson, S.-A. (2002). Characteristics of malingered amnesia: Consequences of withholding vs. distorting information on later memory of a crime event. *Legal and Criminological Psychology*, *7*, 45–61.

Christianson, S.-A. (1992). Remembering emotional events: Potential mechanisms. In S.-A. Christianson (Ed.), *The handbook of emotion and memory: Research and theory* (pp. 307–340). London: Erlbaum.

Christianson, S.-A., & Engelberg, E. (1996). Remembering and forgetting traumatic experiences: A matter of survival. In M. A. Conway (Ed.), *Recovered memories and false memories* (pp. 230–250). Oxford, UK: Oxford University Press.

Christianson, S.-A., & Engelberg, E. (1999). Organization of emotional memories. In T. Dalgleish & M. Power (Eds.), *Handbook of cognition and emotion* (pp. 211–227). Chichester, UK: Wiley.

Conway, M. A. (2001a). Repression revisited. *Nature*, *410*, 319–320.

Conway, M. A. (2001b). Sensory-perceptual episodic memory and its context: Autobiographical memory. *Philosophical Transactions of the Royal Society of London*, *356*, 1–10.

Conway, M. A., Harries, K., Noyes, J., Racsma'ny, M., & Frankish, C. R. (2000). The disruption and dissolution of directed forgetting: Inhibitory control of memory. *Journal of Memory and Language*, *43*, 409–430.

Conway, M. A., & Pleydell-Pearce, C. W. (2000). On the construction of autobiographical memories in a self memory system. *Psychological Review*, *107*, 261–288.

Cox, R., & Barnier, A. J. (2003). Posthypnotic amnesia for a first romantic relationship: Forgetting the entire relationship versus forgetting selected events. *Memory*, *11*, 307–318.

Davis, P. J. (1990). Repression and the inaccessibility of emotional memories. In J. L. Singer (Ed.), *Repression and dissociation: Implications for personality theory, psychopathology, and health* (pp. 387–404). Chicago: University of Chicago Press.

Erdelyi, M. H. (1990). Repression, reconstruction, and defense: History and integration of the psychoanalytic and experimental frameworks. In J. L. Singer (Ed.), *Repression and dissociation: Implications for personality theory, psychopathology, and health* (pp. 1–31). Chicago: University of Chicago Press.

Erdelyi, M. H. (2001). Defense processes can be conscious or unconscious. *American Psychologist*, *56*, 761–762.

Freud, S. (1957). *Repression*. In J. Strachey (Ed. & Trans.) and C. M. Baines (Trans.), *The standard edition of the complete psychological works of Sigmund Freud* (Vol. 14, pp. 147–165). London: Hogarth Press. (Original work published 1915)

Holmes, D. S. (1990). The evidence for repression: An examination of sixty years of research. In J. L. Singer (Ed.), *Repression and dissociation: Implications for personality theory, psychopathology, and health* (pp. 85–102). Chicago: University of Chicago Press.

Jacoby, L. L., Kelley, C., Brown, J., & Jasechko, J. (1989). Becoming famous overnight: Limits on the ability to avoid unconscious influences of the past. *Journal of Personality and Social Psychology*, *56*, 326–338.

Kihlstrom, J. F. (1980). Posthypnotic amnesia for recently learned material: Interactions with "episodic" and "semantic" memory. *Cognitive Psychology*, *12*, 227–251.

Kihlstrom, J. F. (1985). Posthypnotic amnesia and the dissociation of memory. *The Psychology of Learning and Motivation*, *19*, 131–178.

Kihlstrom, J. F. (2002). No need for repression. *Trends in Cognitive Science*, *6*, 502.

Kihlstrom, J. F., & Barnhardt, T. M. (1993). The self-regulation of memory: For better and for worse, with and without hypnosis. In D. M. Wegner & J. Pennebaker (Eds.), *Handbook of mental control* (pp. 88–125). Englewood Cliffs, NJ: Prentice-Hall.

Kihlstrom, J. F., & Schacter, D. L. (1995). Functional disorders of autobiographical memory. In A. Baddeley, B. A. Wilson, & F. Watts (Eds.), *Handbook of memory disorders* (pp. 337–364). London: Wiley.

Koutstaal, W., & Schacter, D. L. (1997). Intentional forgetting and voluntary thought suppression: Two potential methods for coping with childhood trauma. In L. Dickstein & M. B. Riba (Eds.), *American Psychiatric Press review of psychiatry* (Vol. 16, pp. II-79–II-121). Washington, DC: American Psychiatric Press.

MacLeod, C. M. (1998). Directed forgetting. In J. M. Golding & C. M. MacLeod (Eds.), *Intentional forgetting: Interdisciplinary approaches* (pp. 1–57). Mahwah, NJ: Lawrence Erlbaum.

MacLeod, M. (2002). Retrieval-induced forgetting in eyewitness memory: Forgetting as a consequence of remembering. *Applied Cognitive Psychology*, *16*, 135–149.

Macrae, C. N., & MacLeod, M. D. (1999). On recollections lost: When practice makes imperfect. *Journal of Personality and Social Psychology*, *77*, 463–473.

Macrae, C. N., & Roseveare, T. A. (2002). I was always on my mind: The self and temporary forgetting. *Psychonomic Bulletin & Review*, *9*, 611–614.

McAdams, D. P. (2001). The psychology of life stories. *Review of General Psychology*, *5*, 100–122.

McNally, R. J. (2003). *Remembering trauma*. Harvard, MA: Harvard University Press.

Moulin, C. J. A., Perfect, T. J., Conway, M. A., North, A. S., Jones, R. W., & James, N. (2002). Retrieval-induced forgetting in Alzheimer's disease. *Neuropsychologia*, *40*, 862–867.

Myers, L. B., Brewin, C. R., & Power, M. J. (1998). Repressive coping and the directed forgetting of emotional material. *Journal of Abnormal Psychology*, *107*, 141–148.

Perfect, T. J., Moulin, C. J. A., Conway, M. A., & Perry, E. (2002). Assessing the inhibitory account of retrieval-induced forgetting with implicit memory tests. *Journal of Experimental Psychology: Learning, Memory, and Cognition*, *28*, 1111–1119.

Pope, H. G., Hudson, J. I., Bodkin, J. A., & Olivia, P. (1998). Questionable validity of ''dissociative amnesia'' in trauma victims: Evidence from prospective studies. *British Journal of Psychiatry*, *172*, 210–215.

Power, M. J., Dalgleish, T., Claudio, V., Tata, P., & Kentish, J. (2000). The directed forgetting task: Application to emotionally valent material. *Journal of Affective Disorders*, *57*, 147–157.

Schacter, D. L. (1987). Implicit memory: History and current status. *Journal of Experimental psychology: Learning, Memory, and Cognition*, *13*, 501–518.

Shaw, J. S., Bjork, R. A., & Handal, A. (1995). Retrieval-induced forgetting in an eyewitness-memory paradigm. *Psychonomic Bulletin & Review*, *2*, 249–253.

Singer, J. A., & Salovey, P. (1993). *The remembered self.* New York: The Free Press.

Snodgrass, J. G., & Burns, P. M. (1978). The effect of repeated tests on recognition memory for pictures and words. *Bulletin of the Psychonomic Society*, *11*, 263–266.

Spanos, N. P. (1996). *Multiple identities and false memories: A sociocognitive perspective.* Washington, DC: American Psychological Association.

Squire, L. R., & McKee, R. (1992). Influence of prior events on cognitive judgments in amnesia. *Journal of Experimental Psychology: Learning, Memory, and Cognition*, *18*, 106–115.

Tabachnick, B. G., & Fidell, L. S. (1996). *Using multivariate statistics* (3rd ed.). New York: HarperCollins.

Tulving, E., & Pearlstone, Z. (1966). Availability and accessibility of information in memory for words. *Journal of Verbal Learning and Verbal Behavior*, *5*, 381–391.

Weinberger, D. A. (1990). The construct validity of the repressive coping style. In J. L. Singer (Ed.), *Repression and dissociation: Implications for personality theory, psychopathology, and health* (pp. 337–386). Chicago: University of Chicago Press.

Wenzlaff, R. M., & Wegner, D. M. (2000). Thought suppression. *Annual Review of Psychology*, *51*, 59–91.

Wright, D. B., & Nunn, J. A. (2000). Similarities within event clusters in autobiographical memory. *Applied Cognitive Psychology*, *14*, 479–489.

APPENDIX
Experimental stimuli

RIF cue word sets		
A	*B*	*C*
Horrified	Tragedy	Sickness
Patient	Hardworking	Polite
Entertaining	Excitement	Happy

Distribution of cue word sets across RIF experimental phases

	RIF counterbalancing word orders		
Phases	*1*	*2*	*3*
Elicitation	A–C	A–C	A–C
Learning	A–C	A–C	A–C
Retrieval-Practice	A, B	A, C	B, C
Final Recall	A–C	A–C	A–C

	RIF counterbalancing word orders		
Cue word type	*1*	*2*	*3*
Rp	B	A	C
Nrp	C	B	A
Filler	A	C	B

COGNITION AND EMOTION, 2004, *18* (4), 479–493

Inhibiting retrieval of trauma cues in adults reporting histories of childhood sexual abuse

Richard J. McNally, Susan A. Clancy, Heidi M. Barrett, and Holly A. Parker

Harvard University, Cambridge, MA, USA

Are people who report having forgotten their childhood sexual abuse (CSA) characterised by superior ability to inhibit retrieval of disturbing material? To test this hypothesis, we asked adults reporting either repressed, recovered, or continuous memories of CSA or no history of CSA to participate in a directed forgetting experiment (list method). They rated the emotionality of two consecutive lists of trauma-related and positive words. After the first list, the experimenter instructed participants to forget these words, and to continue rating the remaining words. A surprise recall task revealed robust directed forgetting and valence effects: All groups recalled more words from the second list than from the first list, and recalled more trauma words than positive ones. Participants reporting either repressed or recovered memories of CSA did not exhibit superior forgetting of trauma versus positive words relative to the other two groups. Finally, a subsidiary analysis revealed that participants exhibiting a "repressor" coping style (low self-reported anxiety plus high defensiveness) did not exhibit superior directed forgetting of trauma words.

Whether people can accurately recall long-forgotten episodes of childhood sexual abuse (CSA) has been among the most bitter controversies in psychology (McNally, 2003a). Case reports of corroborated sexual abuse suggest that at least some individuals may experience molestation during childhood, not think about it for a long time, and then recall it years later (Cheit, 1998, 1999). Although some theorists have interpreted these reports as evidence that people can repress and then recover memories of overwhelming trauma (i.e.,

Correspondence should be addressed to Richard J. McNally, Department of Psychology, Harvard University, 33 Kirkland Street, Cambridge, MA 02138, USA; e-mail: rjm@wjh.harvard.edu

Preparation of this article was supported by National Institute of Mental Health grant MH61268 awarded to the first author.

http://www.tandf.co.uk/journals/pp/02699931.html DOI:10.1080/02699930341000400

"traumatic amnesia";[1] Brown, Scheflin, & Whitfield, 1999), this interpretation is unwarranted.

There are reasons why these case reports do not provide evidence for *repression* (or dissociation) of *traumatic* memories. Merely because some people do not think about certain experiences for a long period of time does not mean that they have been *unable* to recall them, and it is *inability* to remember that constitutes the essence of repression (McNally, 2003a, pp. 159–228). Indeed, many CSA survivors say that they would have easily remembered their abuse had someone asked them about it during the period of time when they never thought about it (Melchert, 1999). Moreover, people sometimes forget having recalled these experiences during the period of time when they thought they had never thought about them (Schooler, Bendiksen, & Ambadar, 1997). Therefore, retrospective reports of not having thought about one's abuse for many years are not necessarily correct.

One reason why people may forget about their abuse is that the CSA episodes were not experienced as traumatic at the time of their occurrence. For example, many of our participants have told us that episodes of nonviolent abuse (e.g., fondling) were confusing, disgusting, or upsetting, but not "traumatic" in the sense of being life-threatening or terrifying (Clancy & McNally, 2004).[2] Frequently they did not understand it as sexually abusive until after having thought about it much later in adulthood. Accordingly, their failure to think about these experiences do not count as instances of forgetting *trauma*.

The fact that some people seem capable of not thinking about CSA for many years implies individual differences in the ability to put unpleasant events out of mind. Such forms of mental control need not have anything to do with repression or dissociation, but they might explain why some people manage not to think about their CSA. Therefore, do those who report recovering memories of abuse possess superior abilities to forget unwanted material relative to those who report always having remembered their abuse? Can the methods of cognitive psychology detect these abilities in the laboratory?

Clinical researchers have only recently begun to apply experimental methods to investigate memory functioning in people who report recovered memories of CSA (e.g., Clancy, McNally, & Schacter, 1999; Clancy, Schacter, McNally, & Pitman, 2000; McNally, 2003b; McNally, Clancy, & Schacter, 2001). Some

[1] By *traumatic amnesia*, Brown et al. mean an inability to remember a traumatic experience which they attribute to a postulated dissociative or psychic repression mechanism. Traumatic amnesia must not be confused with organic amnesia arising from physical insult to the brain. Nor must it be confused with *psychogenic amnesia*—a syndrome characterised by sudden and complete retrograde memory loss, including loss of personal identity, that cannot be attributed to physical insult to the brain (for a review, see McNally, in press-a).

[2] Of course, to say that molestation is not necessarily traumatic does not in any way justify sexual abuse. As Rind, Tromovitch, and Bauserman (1998) emphasised, merely because sexual abuse does not invariably produce psychiatric disease does not render it morally permissible.

scholars have suggested that directed forgetting methods may be relevant to understanding individual differences in the ability to forget disturbing material (Bjork, 1989; Brewin & Andrews, 1998; Cloitre, Cancienne, Brodsky, Dulit, & Perry, 1996; McNally, in press-b). McNally et al. (2001), for example, used an item-cueing directed forgetting paradigm to investigate forgetting of trauma words in people who either believed they harboured repressed memories of CSA, reported remembering long-forgotten memories of CSA, or reported no history of CSA. Participants viewed a series of words on a computer screen, one at a time. Each word was either trauma-relevant (e.g., *molested*), positive (e.g., *cheerful*), or neutral (e.g., *mailbox*). Immediately after the appearance of each word, participants received an instruction either to remember the word or to forget it. After this encoding phase, participants were asked to recall all words they had seen, irrespective of the original instructions. Individuals who had reportedly forgotten their abuse would seem especially skilled at expelling disturbing material from awareness in this paradigm. Yet contrary to prediction, the repressed and recovered memory groups were not especially adept at forgetting trauma words. Indeed, they recalled to-be-remembered (TBR) words more often than to-be-forgotten (TBF) words, irrespective of the type of word. The results of this study differed from those of another study in which CSA survivors with posttraumatic stress disorder (PTSD) had difficulty recalling positive and neutral words they had been told to remember, while exhibiting excellent memory for trauma words, including those they had been told to forget (McNally, Metzger, Lasko, Clancy, & Pitman, 1998). In this study, 11 of the 12 CSA survivors with PTSD reported always having remembered their abuse. However, in neither of our directed forgetting studies were CSA survivors characterised by superior ability to forget trauma words.

There are at least two mechanisms that might account for directed forgetting effects. Instructions to forget a word may attenuate its encoding, and poor initial encoding might explain why TBF words are not recalled as well as TBR words. Alternatively, TBF words might be encoded into memory, but their retrieval might be inhibited during subsequent recall tests. Our aforementioned directed forgetting experiments involved the item-cueing method—a paradigm yielding results best attributable to differential encoding rather than to retrieval inhibition of encoded material (for reviews, see Golding, in press; Johnson, 1994). That is, recall of TBR words is better than TBF words because participants terminate encoding processes as soon as the forget instruction follows a TBF word, whereas they continue encoding TBR words. Accordingly, the two experiments done by our group provide evidence against the hypothesis that CSA survivors, including those reporting repressed or recovered memories of abuse, are especially skilled at avoiding encoding of trauma words. However, these studies do not test whether these individuals can inhibit retrieval of trauma words that have already been encoded. That is, it is entirely possible that abuse survivors might encode trauma-related cues, but then have difficulty retrieving them later

(Brewin & Andrews, 1998). Indeed, in his influential exposition of the retrieval inhibition concept, Bjork (1989) suggested that retrieval inhibition might figure as a mechanism whereby disturbing memories might be deliberately blocked from awareness.

In the experiment reported here, we used another directed forgetting paradigm—the list method—to test whether CSA survivors, especially those reporting histories of having ''repressed'' their memories of abuse, are characterised by superior retrieval inhibition of trauma words relative to other words and relative to control participants with no reported CSA history. Attenuated recall of TBF items in the list method is best attributed to retrieval inhibition because re-presentation of all words on a recognition test erases the difference in recall between TBR and TBF words (Bjork, 1989; Johnson, 1994). That is, although participants remember more TBR words than TBF words on recall tests, participants remember just as many TBF as TBR words on recognition tests. Presumably, the TBF words get encoded, but are inaccessible until re-exposure to them on the recognition test releases them from inhibition.

Adapting the list method procedure used by Myers, Brewin, and Power (1998), we had participants view and rate a series of words, and then halfway through the list we told them to forget the words they had already seen and to rate the remaining words. Later, they received a surprise free recall test for all words, including those from the first list they had been told to forget. Half of the words in the first list and half of the words in the second list were related to trauma, whereas the remaining words were positive.

We tested several groups of participants. The *repressed memory* group comprised adults who believed they had been sexually abused as children, but who had no explicit autobiographical memory of the abuse. That is, they inferred an abuse history based on diverse ''indicators'' (e.g., brief images interpreted as ''flashbacks'', symptoms of depression). It was impossible for us to determine whether they had, in fact, been abused, but the term ''repressed memory'' does characterise their belief. The *recovered memory* group comprised adults who reported recalling CSA memories after long periods of having not thought about these experiences. [Note that we define a *recovered memory* of sexual abuse purely in descriptive terms as one that has not entered awareness for years. We do not require that the abuse was traumatic (i.e., experienced as life-threatening and overwhelmingly terrifying), nor do we assume that the memory was inaccessible (i.e., repressed, dissociated) during the period when the person did not think about it.] Participants in this group were either unwilling or unable to provide corroboration for the abuse events. This does not, however, mean that their memories of molestation are false.

The *continuous memory* group comprised individuals who reported never having forgotten their abuse. Finally, the *comparison* group comprised individuals who reported never having been sexually abused.

We tested whether participants who reported having forgotten their sexual abuse (recovered and repressed memory groups) exhibit superior ability to inhibit retrieval of trauma-related words relative to positive words and relative to those who had never forgotten their abuse (continuous memory group) or who had never been abused (comparison group). Using a modified version of Myers et al.'s (1998) procedure, we tested whether "repressors"—individuals scoring low on a measure of anxiety but high on a measure of defensiveness (social desirability) exhibit heightened ability to inhibit retrieval of trauma-related words.

METHOD

Participants

To recruit participants, we ran newspaper advertisements that read:

- Were you sexually abused as a child?
- Do you think you might have been sexually abused?
- Do you have no history of childhood sexual abuse?

Individuals responding to the newspaper notices were contacted by Susan A. Clancy, who arranged for the first of three visits. Upon arriving at the laboratory, participants provided written informed consent to participate in the research programme. During the first visit, Dr Clancy conducted a semistructured memory interview that yielded details essential for classifying the participant into one of the groups. Individuals qualifying for either the recovered memory or continuous memory group were asked whether they could furnish corroboration of the abuse. Using the Structured Clinical Interview for DSM-IV (First, Spitzer, Gibbon, & Williams, 1996) and the PTSD Symptom Scale interview (Foa & Tolin, 2000), Dr Clancy assessed for current Axis I mental disorders (Clancy & McNally, 2004).

Continuous memory group. The continuous memory group comprised 72 adults (54 female, 18 male) who reported always having remembered their sexual abuse. Sixteen provided the name of an informant who could corroborate the abuse, and another participant furnished entries from a diary, dating from the time of the abuse, describing her abuse. Dr Clancy spoke to all 16 informants who confirmed the accuracy of the abuse reports.

Seventeen met criteria for CSA-related PTSD, whereas five additional participants had developed PTSD from unrelated traumatic events.

Recovered memory group. The recovered memory group comprised 25 adults (15 female, 10 male) who reported having recovered long-forgotten memories of CSA. Only two participants recollected their abuse during the course of ''recovered memory therapy''. Most of the others were reminded of their abuse after encountering various cues (e.g., television news broadcast about sexual abuse, a magazine article). Seventeen participants reported repeated episodes of molestation. The majority of participants said that they experienced the molestation (usually fondling) as confusing, upsetting, puzzling, and sometimes frightening. None, however, experienced it as traumatic in the sense of being terrifying or life-threatening. None of the participants was either able or willing to furnish corroboration of the abuse.

Two of us (SAC and RJM) independently rated the trauma narrative transcripts on a 4-point credibility scale for 24 participants (The audiotaped transcript for one participant was lost.) Global judgements of credibility were based on several factors [e.g., severity (e.g., violent rape vs. fondling); context of recovery (e.g., ''recovered memory therapy'' vs. encountering a reminder in everyday life); age at abuse (e.g., infancy vs. elementary school age)]. We assigned the same rating for 67% of the cases. When we collapsed the two most credible categories (3 and 4) and the two least credible categories (1 and 2), the percentage agreement was 92%. Both Dr Clancy and Dr McNally gave the highest credibility ratings (a 3 or 4) to 20 participants.

Five met current criteria for CSA-related PTSD.

Repressed memory group. The repressed memory group comprised 33 adults (28 female, 5 male) who believed that they had been sexually abused as children, but who had no autobiographical memories of their abuse. They inferred their abuse histories from diverse indicators such as weight gain, sexual dysfunction, ''body memories'', and depressed mood. Two met criteria for PTSD (unrelated to CSA).

Comparison group. The comparison group comprised 20 adults (11 female, 9 male) who denied ever having been sexually abused as children.

Questionnaires

To characterise our participants further, we asked them to complete the following questionnaires. The Dissociative Experiences Scale (DES: Bernstein & Putnam, 1986) measured dissociative symptoms (e.g., ''spacing out'', memory lapses); the Absorption Scale (Tellegen & Atkinson, 1974) measured proneness to become engaged in imaginative experiences—a correlate of fantasy proneness; the Beck Depression Inventory (BDI: Beck & Steer, 1987) measured depressive symptoms; the short form of the Manifest Anxiety Scale (MAS: Bendig, 1956) measured trait anxiety; the Marlowe-Crowne Social Desirability Scale (MC: Crowne & Marlowe, 1964) measured defensiveness; and the Shipley scales provided measures of verbal and nonverbal cognitive ability (Zachary, 1991). We also recorded age and years of education.

The means and standard deviations for these variables are shown in Table 1. As confirmed by analyses of variance (ANOVAs), the groups did not differ (*ps* > .05) in terms of age, education, or defensiveness (MC). Significant effects emerged for the other variables, and we conducted post hoc contrasts (least-significant differences method) to explore these further. We report only significant contrasts ($p < .05$). The continuous, recovered, and repressed memory groups scored higher than the comparison group on the DES and the Absorption scale. As reflected in their MAS scores, the repressed memory group reported more anxiety symptoms than did the other groups, and the continuous memory group reported more symptoms than did the comparison group. Both the repressed and continuous memory groups reported more symptoms of depression than did the comparison group. Both the comparison and repressed memory groups scored higher on measures of both verbal and nonverbal cognitive ability than did the continuous memory group.

TABLE 1
Mean for demographic and psychometric data

	Group					
	Comparison	*Continuous*	*Recovered*	*Repressed*		
Variable	*M*	*M*	*M*	*M*	*F*	*p*
Age	36.0	37.9	41.3	40.8	1.2	.32
(3, 153)	(13.2)	(10.6)	(15.4)	(10.6)		
Education	15.0	14.8	14.8	15.8	1.4	.24
(3, 153)	(1.7)	(2.3)	(2.6)	(1.9)		
DES	8.1	17.7	16.7	21.3	4.1	.01
(3, 147)	(7.4)	(13.9)	(11.0)	(14.9)		
Absorption	13.1	18.2	19.6	18.1	3.3	.02
(3, 145)	(7.6)	(7.0)	(7.3)	(6.8)		
BDI	7.0	14.7	12.1	17.2	4.6	.00
(3, 146)	(7.2)	(10.5)	(8.0)	(11.0)		
MAS	5.8	9.4	8.9	12.4	6.5	.00
(3, 146)	(5.6)	(5.5)	(4.7)	(5.1)		
MC	15.8	14.6	14.9	14.2	.3	.80
(3, 146)	(7.3)	(5.4)	(5.2)	(5.3)		
Shipley-V	33.8	30.8	33.4	34.1	3.3	.02
(3, 148)	(4.1)	(6.8)	(5.1)	(2.9)		
Shipley-NV	16.4	14.2	15.6	16.3	3.2	.02
(3, 149)	(3.1)	(3.9)	(3.0)	(3.5)		

Note: Because of missing data, degrees of freedom vary. The degrees of freedom for each ANOVA are in parentheses underneath the variable title. Standard deviations are in parentheses underneath the means. DES = Dissociative Experiences Scale; BDI = Beck Depression Inventory; MAS = short form of the Manifest Anxiety Scale; MC = Marlowe-Crowne Social Desirability Scale; Shipley-V = verbal scale; Shipley-NV = nonverbal scale.

In addition to using questionnaires to characterise the groups, we also used the MAS and the MC to classify participants as "repressors" and "nonrepressors". Following Myers et al. (1998), we classified a participant as a "repressor" if he/she scored 8 or lower on the MAS ($M = 4.0$) and 17 or higher on the MC ($M = 21.3$). Thirty-two participants qualified as repressors. The numbers of participants from each group and the percentage of each group qualifying were as follows: repressed memory group ($n = 5$, 15%); recovered memory group ($n = 7$, 28%); continuous memory group ($n = 15$, 21%); comparison group ($n = 5$, 25%). Participants scoring 9 or higher on the MAS ($M = 14.2$) and 16 or lower on the MC ($M = 10.8$) were designated as "nonrepressors". Fifty-five participants qualified as nonrepressors. The numbers of participants from each group and the percentage of each group qualifying were as follows: repressed memory group ($n = 15$, 46%); recovered memory group ($n = 8$, 32%); continuous memory group ($n = 30$, 42%); comparison group ($n = 3$, 15%). The remaining participants who met either repressor or nonrepressor criteria for only the MAS or the MC were excluded from these analyses.

Materials and procedure

Each participant saw two consecutive lists of words. Each word appeared one at a time on a Gateway 386 personal computer, as programmed by MicroExperimental Laboratory (MEL; Schneider, 1988). Each word appeared for 3 s at centre screen in white lower case letters against a blue background. The interstimulus interval was 5 s. Three neutral (filler) words preceded the first list: *sensible*, *quick*, and *moderate*. Each experimental list comprised 10 positive (P) and 10 trauma-related (T) words, all drawn from our previous research on memory in sexual abuse survivors (McNally et al., 1998). List A consisted of *shock* (T), *assault* (T), *secure* (P), *steady* (P), *reassured* (P), *humiliated* (T), *incest* (T), *molested* (T), *elation* (P), *relieved* (P), *abused* (T), *crime* (T), *confident* (P), *cheerful* (P), *carefree* (P), *nightmare* (T), *pleasure* (P), *scream* (T), *worthless* (T), and *healthy* (P). List B consisted of *sincere* (P), *rape* (T), *charming* (P), *terror* (T), *brutal* (T), *outgoing* (P), *affection* (P), *tortured* (T), *victim* (T), *painful* (T), *shame* (T), *happiness* (P), *easygoing* (P), *penis* (T), *violence* (T), *friendly* (P), *ecstasy* (P), *sociable* (P), *celebrate* (P), and *semen* (T). The words appeared in a random order within each list. The positive and trauma word groups did not differ in terms of their mean frequency of usage in American English (Francis & Kučera, 1982) or in terms of mean word length. We counterbalanced Lists A and B within each group (i.e., List A was presented before List B for half of each group, whereas the order was reversed for the remaining participants).

The experimenter read the following instructions to the participant. (All the instructions appeared on the computer screen as the experimenter read them to the participant):

> You will be asked to rate a series of words in terms of their emotional meaning. Each word will appear on this computer screen for 3 seconds. When the word appears, you should rate its emotional meaning on this seven-point scale.
>
> | Very negative | | | | | | Very positive |
> |---|---|---|---|---|---|---|
> | −3 | −2 | −1 | 0 | +1 | +2 | +3 |
>
> As you can see, the scale ranges from −3 (very negative) to +3 (very positive). If the word has no emotional meaning for you, you should rate it a 0. A 5 second delay will occur after each word appears. I will ask you to say out loud what your rating is, and I will record it on this sheet. Any questions?

If the participant had no questions, he/she pressed the space bar to initiate the program. After the first list was presented, the participant received the following instructions:

> What you have done so far is practice. You can forget about those words. I will now show you the actual set of test words that I want you to rate in the same way you did for the practice words.

Although the participant was directed to forget the first list of words, he/she was not directed to remember the second list. For ease of exposition, though, we refer to the first list of words as TBF items, and the second list as TBR items. After the participant completed the second list, the experimenter then presented the next "task" to the participant: A filler task consisting of a series of 84 easy addition and subtraction problems (e.g., 10+81 = ?). The experimenter said:

> Please complete as many of these mathematical equations as you can before I ask you to stop.

The participant was allowed 3 minutes to complete these problems before the experimenter presented the free recall task by saying:

> Please write down as many words as you can remember seeing from BOTH lists.

The participant was given 5 minutes to recall the words.

RESULTS

A 4 (Group: comparison vs. continuous vs. recovered vs. repressed memory) × 2 (Instructions: TBR vs. TBF) × 2 (Valence: trauma vs. positive) ANOVA yielded significant effects for Group, $F(3, 146) = 4.76$, $p = .003$, Instructions, $F(1, 146) = 40.53$, $p < .001$, and Valence, $F(1, 146) = 75.21$, $p < .001$. Post-hoc contrasts (least significant differences method) indicated that both the comparison group and the recovered memory group recalled more words than did the continuous memory group; that participants recalled more TBR words than TBF

TABLE 2
Mean number (and standard deviations) of words recalled as a function of group, instructions, and word type

Instructions	*Trauma*	*Positive*
Comparison group (n = 20)		
Remember	4.20 (2.02)	3.65 (2.39)
Forget	3.55 (1.70)	2.25 (1.55)
Continuous memory group (n = 72)		
Remember	3.58 (1.68)	2.26 (1.48)
Forget	2.76 (1.52)	1.51 (1.40)
Recovered memory group (n = 25)		
Remember	4.24 (1.42)	3.48 (1.96)
Forget	3.08 (1.58)	2.08 (1.63)
Repressed memory group (n = 33)		
Remember	3.64 (1.67)	2.94 (1.94)
Forget	3.24 (1.58)	1.85 (1.30)

Note: Possible range of scores for each cell: 0 to 10 words recalled.

TABLE 3
Mean number (and standard deviations) of words recalled as a function of repressor versus nonrepressor status, instructions, and word type

Instructions	*Trauma*	*Positive*
Repressors (n = 32)		
Remember	3.47 (1.67)	2.22 (1.31)
Forget	3.13 (1.58)	1.81 (1.36)
Nonrepressors (n = 56)		
Remember	4.04 (1.63)	2.91 (1.92)
Forget	3.13 (1.65)	1.84 (1.25)

Note: Possible range of scores for each cell: 0 to 10 words recalled.

words; and that participants recalled more trauma than positive words. None of the interactions was significant.

A 2 (Group: repressor vs. nonrepressor) × 2 (Instructions: TBR vs. TBF) × 2 (Valence: trauma vs. positive) revealed that participants recalled more TBR words than TBF words: Instructions, $F(1, 86) = 12.68$, $p = .001$, and that participants recalled more trauma than positive words: Valence, $F(1, 86) = 81.81$, $p < .001$. There were no other significant effects, *ps* > .11.

Additional analyses

Because Cloitre et al. (1996) reported that elevated dissociation scores predicted better memory for TBR words (positive, neutral, and negative combined), we computed correlations between DES scores and recall scores. None of the correlations was significant. The *rs*(132) were: TBR-trauma = −.03; TBR-positive = .09; TBF-trauma = −.01; TBF-positive = −.04. The DES correlated with the Absorption scale, $r(132) = .56$, $p = .0001$. But as with the DES, none of the correlations between Absorption and word recall measures was significant.

Because all groups recalled more trauma words than positive words, we tested whether trauma words were rated higher than positive words in terms of absolute levels of emotionality. Perhaps participants rated trauma words as more personally negative than they rated positive words positive. To test this hypothesis, we submitted the mean (absolute) emotionality ratings of the words to a 4 (Group: comparison vs. continuous vs. recovered vs. repressed memory) × 2 (Instructions: TBR vs. TBF) × 2 (Valence: trauma vs. positive) ANOVA. None of the effects was significant, *Fs* > .10, including the effect of valence: $F(1, 120) = 0.01$, $p = .94$. (Missing data from some subjects lowered the *df* for the error term.)

DISCUSSION

All groups exhibited robust directed forgetting effects as evinced by superior recall of TBR words than TBF words. Contrary to prediction, neither group with reported histories of having forgotten abuse exhibited superior forgetting of trauma words versus positive words. Moreover, all groups exhibited better recall for trauma words than positive words. The fact that even the comparison group exhibited superior recall of trauma words is likely attributable to the especially shocking salience of these words (e.g., *incest*, *rape*) compared to the negative words in some previous directed forgetting experiments (e.g., *criticism*, *lonely*, Cloitre et al., 1996; *thoughtless*, *unhappy*, Myers et al., 1998). That is, although trauma and positive words did not differ on absolute values of personal emotional significance—all participants tend to give +3 ratings to words like *elation* and *happiness* and −3 ratings to words like *rape* and *tortured*—the shocking salience of the latter may nevertheless render them especially memorable for anyone, regardless of his/her abuse history.

There are several possible explanations for the failure of groups reporting either repressed or recovered memories of CSA to exhibit the predicted superior ability to inhibit retrieval of trauma words. First, contrary to certain theorists (e.g., Terr, 1991), people sexually abused as children may not possess superior ability to forget trauma cues. Indeed, our previous research suggests that abuse victims with PTSD exhibit impairment in the ability to forget trauma words (McNally et al., 1998). Second, at least some participants reporting repressed or recovered memories of CSA may not have been abused. Third, contrary to speculation (Brewin & Andrews, 1998; Cloitre et al., 1996; McNally, in press-b), experimental directed forgetting paradigms may fail to engage the relevant inhibitory mechanisms that enable abuse victims to avoid thinking about their early adverse experiences for many years. For example, the time-frame of encoding, forgetting, and retrieval is less than a hour, not a matter of years. On the other hand, in defence of the relevance of these paradigms, Moulds and Bryant (2002, in press) reported enhanced directed forgetting of trauma cues in patients with acute stress disorder.

In contrast to Myers et al. (1998), we did not find that ''repressors'' exhibited superior directed forgetting of negative information. There are several possible reasons for the differences between our results and theirs. Although we used their criteria for defining repressor and nonrepressor groups, ours included older participants, many of whom had been abused. Moreover, our word rating task differed from theirs. Myers et al. had participants rate words in terms of self-relevance, whereas we had them rate words in terms of emotionality. For two reasons, we did not use adjective self-ratings. First, there are very few words that are related to sexual abuse trauma, even when one defines it broadly, including words, such as *tortured* and *semen*. Therefore, it would be difficult to come up with enough adjectives to enable us to use a self-referent encoding task. Hence, we used a mix of nouns and adjectives. Second, the aims of our respective studies differed. For example, we were concerned with the ability of survivors to suppress material related to their abuse, not with the ability to suppress negative material relevant to the self.

Perhaps most importantly, their repressor participants differ markedly from our participants who believe they harbour repressed memories of sexual abuse. In this study as well as in our previous research (McNally, Clancy, Schacter, & Pitman, 2000), repressed memory participants reported high levels of emotional distress, whereas ''repressors'' report low levels of distress.

To date, clinical studies involving the list method have been characterised by a potential limitation: The absence of a remember-remember condition (Moulds & Bryant, in press; Myers et al., 1998; the present experiment). That is, the list receiving remember instructions is always the most recent list, thereby raising the possibility that superior recall of TBR words versus TBF words is attributable not to inhibition, but to a recency effect favouring TBR words. To test this, researchers would have to include a control group whereby participants are told to remember the first list as well as the second list. On the other hand, a failure to include a remember-remember group may not fatally compromise interpretation of the data. For example, the well-known serial position effect in verbal learning implies that not only the most recent words should be easily recalled, but also the earliest words from the first list. The inverted-U pattern implies that memory should be weakest for the words in the middle of the experiment (i.e., the final words in list one and the early words in list two).

Our correlational analyses failed to uncover significant predictors of directed forgetting. If one assumes that dissociative tendencies tap an ability to block awareness of disturbing material, then scores on the DES should have correlated with inhibition of trauma words. But these null findings are in accord with our previous study in which DES scores were not significantly related to directed forgetting of trauma words (McNally et al., 2001).

In summary, we found no evidence of superior ability to inhibit retrieval of words related to trauma in people reporting either repressed or recovered memories of sexual abuse. Although directed forgetting methods cannot determine whether people were really abused or whether they had forgotten their abuse, these paradigms may illuminate mechanisms that might figure in such processes.

REFERENCES

Beck, A. T., & Steer, R. A. (1987). *Beck Depression Inventory manual*. San Antonio, TX: Psychological Corporation.

Bendig, A. W. (1956). The development of a short form of the Manifest Anxiety Scale. *Journal of Consulting Psychology*, *20*, 384.

Bernstein, E. M., & Putnam, F. W. (1986). Development, reliability, and validity of a dissociation scale. *Journal of Nervous and Mental Disease*, *174*, 727–735.

Bjork, R. A. (1989) Retrieval inhibition as an adaptive mechanism in human memory. In H. L. Roediger III & F. I. M. Craik (Eds.), *Varieties of memory and consciousness: Essays in honor of Endel Tulving* (pp. 309–330). Hillsdale, NJ: Erlbaum.

Brewin, C. R., & Andrews, B. (1998). Recovered memories of trauma: Phenomenology and cognitive mechanisms. *Clinical Psychology Review*, *18*, 949–970.

Brown, D., Scheflin, A. W., & Whitfield, C. L. (1999). Recovered memories: The current weight of the evidence in science and in the courts. *Journal of Psychiatry and Law*, *27*, 5–156.

Cheit, R. E. (1998). Consider this, skeptics of recovered memory. *Ethics and Behavior*, *8*, 141–160.

Cheit, R. E. (1999). Junk skepticism and recovered memory: A reply to Piper. *Ethics and Behavior*, *9*, 295–318.

Clancy, S. A., & McNally, R. J. (2004). *Recovered memories of childhood sexual abuse: Forgetting as a consequence of voluntary suppression*. Manuscript submitted for publication.

Clancy, S. A., McNally, R. J., & Schacter, D. L. (1999). Effects of guided imagery on memory distortion in women reporting recovered memories of childhood sexual abuse. *Journal of Traumatic Stress*, *12*, 559–569.

Clancy, S. A., Schacter, D. L., McNally, R. J., & Pitman, R. K. (2000). False recognition in women reporting recovered memories of sexual abuse. *Psychological Science*, *11*, 26–31.

Cloitre, M., Cancienne, J., Brodsky, B., Dulit, R., & Perry, S. W. (1996). Memory performance among women with parental abuse histories: Enhanced directed forgetting or directed remembering? *Journal of Abnormal Psychology*, *105*, 204–211.

Crowne, D. P., & Marlowe, D. A. (1960). A new scale of social desirability independent of psychopathology. *Journal of Consulting Psychology*, *24*, 349–354.

First, M. B., Spitzer, R. L., Gibbon, M., & Williams, J. B. W. (1996). *Structured clinical interview for DSM-IV axis I disorders.* New York: Biometrics Research Department, New York State Psychiatric Institute.

Foa, E. B., & Tolin, D. F. (2000). Comparison of the PTSD Symptom Scale-Interview Version and the Clinician-Administered PTSD Scale. *Journal of Traumatic Stress*, *13*, 181–191.

Francis, W. N., & Kučera, H. (1982). *Frequency analysis of English usage.* Boston, MA: Houghton Mifflin.

Golding, J. M. (in press). Understanding directed forgetting. In A. Wenzel & D. C. Rubin (Eds.), *Cognitive methods and their application to clinical research.* Washington, DC: American Psychological Association Press.

Johnson, H. M. (1994). Processes of successful intentional forgetting. *Psychological Bulletin*, *116*, 274–292.

McNally, R. J. (2003a). *Remembering trauma.* Cambridge, MA: Belknap Press/Harvard University Press.

McNally, R. J. (2003b). Recovering memories of trauma: A view from the laboratory. *Current Directions in Psychological Science*, *12*, 32–35.

McNally, R. J. (in press-a). The science and folklore of traumatic amnesia. *Clinical Psychology: Science and Practice.*

McNally, R. J. (in press-b). Directed forgetting of emotional material. In A. Wenzel & D. C. Rubin (Eds.), *Cognitive methods and their application to clinical research.* Washington, DC: American Psychological Association Press.

McNally, R. J., Clancy, S. A., Schacter, D. L., & Pitman, R. K. (2000). Personality profiles, dissociation, and absorption in women reporting repressed, recovered, or continuous memories of childhood sexual abuse. *Journal of Consulting and Clinical Psychology*, *68*, 1033–1037.

McNally, R. J., Clancy, S. A., & Schacter, D. L. (2001). Directed forgetting of trauma cues in adults reporting repressed or recovered memories of childhood sexual abuse. *Journal of Abnormal Psychology*, *110*, 151–156.

McNally, R. J., Metzger, L. J., Lasko, N. B., Clancy, S. A., & Pitman, R. K. (1998). Directed forgetting of trauma cues in adult survivors of childhood sexual abuse with and without posttraumatic stress disorder. *Journal of Abnormal Psychology*, *107*, 596–601.

Melchert, T. P. (1999). Relations among childhood memory, a history of abuse, dissociation, and repression. *Journal of Interpersonal Violence*, *14*, 1172–1192.

Moulds, M. L., & Bryant, R. A. (2002). Directed forgetting in acute stress disorder. *Journal of Abnormal Psychology*, *111*, 175–179.

Moulds, M. L., & Bryant, R. A. (in press). Retrieval inhibition of traumatic stimuli in acute stress disorder. *Journal of Traumatic Stress.*

Myers, L. B., Brewin, C. R., & Power, M. J. (1998). Repressive coping and the directed forgetting of emotional material. *Journal of Abnormal Psychology*, *107*, 141–148.

Rind, B., Tromovitch, P., & Bauserman, R. (1998). A meta-analytic examination of assumed properties of child sexual abuse using college samples. *Psychological Bulletin*, *124*, 22–53.

Schneider, W. (1988). Micro Experimental Laboratory: An integrated system for IBM PC compatibles. *Behavior Research Methods, Instrumentation, and Computers*, *20*, 206–217.

Schooler, J. W., Bendiksen, M., & Ambadar, Z. (1997). Taking the middle line: Can we accommodate both fabricated and recovered memories of sexual abuse? In M. A. Conway (Ed.), *Recovered memories and false memories* (pp. 251–292). Oxford, UK: Oxford University Press.

Tellegen, A., & Atkinson, G. (1974). Openness to absorbing and self-altering experiences (''absorption''), a trait related to hypnotic susceptibility. *Journal of Abnormal Psychology*, *83*, 268–277.

Terr, L. C. (1991). Childhood trauma: An outline and overview. *American Journal of Psychiatry*, *148*, 10–20.

Zachary, R. A. (1991). *Shipley Institute of Living Scale* (revised). Los Angeles: Western Psychological Services.

COGNITION AND EMOTION, 2004, *18* (4), 495–511

To forget or not to forget: What do repressors forget and when do they forget?

Lynn B. Myers
University College London, UK

Nazanin Derakshan
University of Leeds, UK

Using a directed forgetting task, we tested the hypothesis that repressors would be superior to nonrepressors in forgetting negative experimental material. Consistent with previous studies, there was an overall directed forgetting effect, with significantly more to-be-remembered (TBR) material recalled than to-be-forgotten material (TBF). As predicted, there were no recall differences for negative words in a control condition without the instruction to forget. Repressors compared to nonrepressors forgot more negatively valenced words in the TBF set only in a private condition where they had to rate words for self-descriptiveness but not for other-descriptiveness and not in the public condition. These results suggest that repressors have an enhanced capability for employing retrieval inhibition in certain conditions (e.g., private conditions), but not public conditions when under evaluation. The results support the notion of repressors as self-deceivers rather than impression managers.

There is a large body of evidence indicating that a group of low trait anxiety individuals who exhibit a repressive coping style (repressors) exhibit an avoidant processing style (see Myers, 2000, for a review) and have deficits regarding negative memories (e.g., Myers & Brewin, 1995, 1994; Myers, Brewin, & Power, 1998).

The classification of repressors using a measure of trait anxiety, such as the trait scale of the State-Trait Anxiety Inventory (STAI; Spielberger, Gorsuch, Lushene, Vagg, & Jacobs, 1983), and a measure of defensiveness, such as the Marlowe-Crowne Social Desirability Scale (Crowne & Marlowe, 1964) was

Correspondence should be addressed to Dr Lynn B Myers, Unit of Health Psychology, Centre for Behavioural and Social Sciences in Medicine, University College London, Wolfson Building, 48 Riding House Street, London, UK; e-mail: l.myers@ucl.ac.uk.

This research was supported, in part, by the Royal Society Dorothy Hodgkin Fellowship awarded to Naz Derakshan.

http://www.tandf.co.uk/journals/pp/02699931.html DOI:10.1080/02699930341000419

developed by Weinberger, Schwartz, and Davidson (1979). They identified four groups according to their coping styles: *Repressors* (low anxiety-high defensiveness, REP), *low anxious* (low anxiety-low defensiveness, LA), *high anxious* (high anxiety-low defensiveness, HA), and *defensive high anxious* (high anxiety-high defensiveness, DHA). Under stressful conditions, repressors report low levels of distress but are physiologically and behaviourally very reactive (e.g., Asendorpf & Scherer, 1983; Benjamins, Schuurs, & Hoogstraten, 1994; Derakshan & Eysenck, 1997, 1999, 2001a, 2002b; Weinberger et al., 1979).

A series of studies indicated that repressors have limited accessibility of both childhood and more recent memories (Davies, 1987; Davis & Schwartz, 1987; Myers, Brewin, & Power, 1992). For example, Myers et al. (1992) found that repressors compared to nonrepressors recalled significantly fewer negative (but not positive) memories and took longer to retrieve negative memories (but not positive) in cued recall tasks.

Later research has indicated that repressors possess an information-processing style that affects more than the retrieval of their own personal histories. For example, Boden and Baumeister (1997) found that repressors were faster at recalling happy memories after watching an unpleasant film than watching a neutral film, whereas nonrepressors exhibited the opposite effect. In a study where participants were asked to intentionally learn a story containing positive and negative information and were asked to relate it to themselves, repressors recalled significantly fewer negative phrases than nonrepressors whereas there was no difference in the recall of positive or neutral phrases (Myers & Brewin, 1995).

The mechanism by which such material may be forgotten was investigated in two experiments by Myers et al. (1998) using the directed forgetting paradigm (see also McNally et al., this issue). In the directed forgetting task, stimuli such as words or sentences, are presented. There are, typically, two methods used to designate some material as to-be-forgotten (TBF) and some material as to-be-remembered (TBR). In the list method midway through presentation of the list, participants are instructed to forget the first half of the list and remember the second half of the list. In the word method stimuli are designated TBF or TBR by instructions given directly after individual presentation of each stimulus. Using either method, participants given a surprise recall test of the entire set of stimuli recall fewer of the TBF set than of the TBR set. The directed forgetting paradigm has been widely used to investigate individual differences including studies of people with borderline personality disorder (Korfine & Hooley, 2000), depression (Power, Dalgleish, Claudio, Tata, & Kentish, 2000), acute stress disorder (Moulds & Bryant, 2002), and obsessive-compulsive disorder (Tolin, Hamlin, & Foa, 2002).

Originally, theories of directed forgetting have tended to emphasise selective remembering rather than selective forgetting. Bjork (1970, 1972), for example, argued that two interrelated processes operating at encoding can account for the directed forgetting effect. According to this view, participants engaged in selective rehearsal, and devoted all rehearsal after the *forget* instruction to the TBR items. In addition, participants group TBR items in memory in such a way that functionally separates them from the items that they are to forget. However, later studies have indicated that these two explanations are not sufficient. For example, Jongeward, Woodward, and Bjork (1975) gave participants a demanding task and instructed them to devote all their rehearsal activities to the current set of words, hence allowing little if any time for differential processing of TBR versus TBF words. When participants were asked to recall TBR words only, participants still differentiated the two sets of words.

Geiselman, Bjork, and Fishman (1983) therefore postulated a further process to take place during directed forgetting. They hypothesised that the *forget* cue inhibits routes to the TBF items, resulting in retrieval inhibition. To test this hypothesis, Geiselman et al. (1983) developed a related paradigm involving a mixture of intentional and incidental learning. The innovation was that some material throughout the list was learned intentionally, while other material was learned incidentally, via a pleasantness judgement task, and was therefore not explicitly associated with the *forget* cue. Hence, whatever effect the *forget* instruction may have had on the retention of the incidental items, it was extremely unlikely to have been due to selective rehearsal, as these stimuli were not intended to be remembered. The recall of the incidentally presented items was then compared to that of intentionally learned items that were to be forgotten. With this paradigm, a midlist instruction to forget the first half of the list was found to reduce later recall of items learned incidentally as well as those learned intentionally. In addition, there was no difference in a recognition task. The authors concluded that these results could only be explained by postulating that a cue to forget inhibits access to the TBF items. Because recognition performance was unimpaired, they concluded that the inhibition induced via the *forget* cue took the form of retrieval inhibition.

Myers et al. (1998) postulated that repressors would be better at forgetting negative words which had been rated for self-descriptiveness. In order to test the retrieval inhibition hypothesis, the list method was used. A task solely involving incidental recall was used to guard against the possibility that participants high in social desirability would be more motivated to learn or forget if this was part of the task instructions. In two experiments, repressors forgot more negatively valenced words in the TBF set than nonrepressors, suggesting that repressors have an enhanced capability for employing retrieval inhibition. There were no differences in recall of TBF positive words and both TBR negative and TBR positive words. These experiments provided additional evidence that repressors have poorer recall, not only for negative autobiographical memories, but also for negative experimental material.

The current experiment used the directed forgetting paradigm to replicate and extend the Myers et al. (1998) experiments. In those experiments, it is not clear whether the self-referent dimension of the task (rating adjectives for self-descriptiveness) was crucial in obtaining selective forgetting. Although it is probable that repressors' avoidance of negative affect may be limited to negative material related to self (see Myers, 2000 for a review), this has not been empirically tested using the directed forgetting paradigm. In the current directed forgetting experiment, repressors and nonrepressors rated adjectives for self and other descriptiveness. In addition, a condition was added where words were rated without the ''forget'' instruction, to clarify that this instruction is important for any enhanced directed forgetting effect exhibited by repressors.

A second variable that affects repressors' performance on cognitive tasks is whether they operate in a private or public setting (e.g., Baumeister & Cairns, 1992; Derakshan & Lilja, 2003; Newton & Contrada, 1992). Baumeister and Cairns (1992) tested repressors and nonrepressors in a private condition (they remained anonymous) and a public condition (they were asked for their name and other personal details). Participants were tested in pairs with trait anxiety/defensiveness scales administered by computer. After they had completed the scales the computer produced a bogus personality profile supposedly based on the former test. In the private condition, participants were reassured that no one would ever see the profile and that it was data to investigate broad statistical trends. In the public condition participants were told that these data would be shown to their experimental partners. All participants were left alone to read their profile at their chosen speed. There were two supposed profiles, one good and one bad. Participants were then told the profiles were bogus and to write down as many adjectives from them as they could remember.

Repressors who received threatening feedback privately spent the least amount of time reading it, whereas repressors who received the same feedback publicly spent a long time reading it. They also spent less time reading the unfavourable compared to favourable evaluation. Nonrepressors were unaffected by the favourability of the evaluation or the public nature of the situation. It would appear that in the private condition, repressors used an avoidant strategy to dismiss negative information concerning self. However, this strategy was not used in the public condition. The current experiment explored whether there would be similar findings in a directed forgetting task and it was hypothesised that repressors would show enhanced directed forgetting for self-referent negative words in a private condition but not a public condition.

One of the major difficulties with this area of research is the fact that the trait anxiety/defensiveness method depends on categorising people into groups based on their location along two dimensions. For example, various studies identify their participants at the beginning of the study by screening a large number of potential participants and choosing extreme scorers on trait anxiety and defensiveness to define repressors, low anxious, high anxious, and (possibly) defensive high anxious groups (e.g., Asendorpf & Scherer, 1983; Derakshan & Eysenck, 1997, 1998, 1999; Myers & Brewin, 1994, 1995), while others use median splits (e.g., Jensen, 1987; Niaura, Herbert, McMahon & Somerville, 1992). However, there is a potential problem using this latter method, as median splits may allow borderline repressors to be included in the analyses, whereas using extreme-scoring participants omits such participants and allows for more confidence that individuals defined as repressors are truly repressors (see Myers, 2000). To investigate this dilemma, both median and quartile splits were used to compare the performance of repressors and nonrepressors in the current experiment.

Therefore the main hypothesis was that repressors compared to nonrepressors will forget more negative words in the TBF set when the words are related to self but not other. This will only be found in the private condition. It was also investigated as to whether results will be clear using median splits on trait anxiety/ defensiveness, or whether it was necessary to use quartile splits.

METHOD

Participants

A total of 236 undergraduate students from the University of Leeds participated in this study. There were 78 males and 158 females, mean age 23.4, age range of 18–26 years. Participants were volunteers who responded to a university-wide e-mail and posters used for recruiting participants for psychological experiments.

Median splits on trait anxiety (STAI) and defensiveness (Marlowe-Crowne) initially classified participants into four groups: repressor (REP, low anxiety-high defensiveness), low anxious (LA, low anxiety-low defensiveness), high anxious (HA, high anxiety-low defensiveness), and defensive high anxious groups (DHA, high anxiety-high defensiveness). Median splits for STAI and MC were 44 and 14, respectively. This resulted in 59 repressors, 54 low anxious, 75 high anxious, and 45 defensive high anxious participants.

Participants were subsequently divided into quartile splits on the two measures. Quartile splits for the STAI were 36 (lower bound) and 51 (upper bound), and for the Marlowe-Crowne were 9 (lower bound) and 18 (upper bound). These cut-off points are consistent with previous studies of Derakshan and Eysenck (1997, 1998, 1999). This classification resulted in 27 repressor, 16 low anxious, 31 high anxious, and 19 defensive high anxious participants.

It should be noted that in some recent studies on repressive coping the trait anxiety and repressive-defensiveness scales have been treated as continuous measures and analysed using hierarchical regression analysis (e.g., Mendolia, 2002). The preference of classification using cut-off points to continuous measures has been a methodological concern that has mainly involved the relationship between the two measures of anxiety and defensiveness that ranges between a small to a moderate negative correlation. However, it has been shown that either method would result in comparable findings given the appropriate power and sample size (e.g., Mendolia, 2002). In the current investigation, the correlation between anxiety and defensiveness was $r = -.128$, $p = .051$. This supported our decision for treating the two measures as somewhat orthogonal using a mixed design analysis of variance. This is an important issue to consider as the interaction effect of trait anxiety × defensiveness would lead to a clearer interpretation of a repressor effect that could be attributable to low levels of anxiety/high levels of defensiveness rather than overlapping or additive main effects of anxiety or defensiveness.

Design

The design of the current investigation was a 2 × 2 × 2 × 2 completely randomised between-subject design, with conditions of forget/nonforget, public/private, and trait anxiety (low, high), and defensiveness (low, high) as the between-subject factors.

Description of computer task. Participants received the following standardised instructions on the screen: ''In this experiment you will be taking part in a self-perception task. You will be presented with a number of words and will be asked to rate each word on a 1 to 4 point scale, for how descriptive of yourself, or how descriptive of an average fellow student, the same sex and age as you, the word would be with (1 = not at all descriptive, and 4 = very descriptive). You will have a limited time of 10 seconds for rating the word. Once you enter your rating, the task will proceed onto the next word''.

Throughout the task the words were presented in a random order, except for the three practice words (not included in the main task) that always came first. One of two reference questions would appear on the screen: ''How descriptive of yourself is this word?'', or: ''How descriptive is this word of an average fellow student, same age and sex as you?''. The word to be rated appeared below the question and below that appeared the rating scale. The rating scale was from 1–4 (1 = not at all descriptive to 4 = very descriptive). Participants were asked to make their responses by clicking (with the mouse) on one of the four rating buttons that best described their response. When a response was made the program moved on to the next trial. If after 10 seconds no response was made, then the program automatically moved onto the next trial.

Private and public conditions. In the private condition the blind was pulled down over the two-way mirror in order to emphasise privacy. At the beginning of the experiment, just before the main experimental task, in the private condition, participants received the following ''privacy statement'': ''Note that all your responses in this rating task will be kept absolutely confidential and will not be used for any purpose other than the current experiment''.

In the public condition the two-way mirror was revealed and participants received the following statement before the experiment began: "Note that while performing on the rating task a lecturer in the room next door will be observing this session through the one-way mirror. This is for methodological purposes". The identity of the experimenter remained anonymous.

Forgetting instructions. In the private and public conditions that involved directed forgetting instructions, half way through the rating task, participants received the following instructions on the screen: "What you have done so far has been practice. You can forget about those words. You will now be shown the actual set of words that you are asked to rate for self-descriptiveness and other-descriptiveness, in the same way as you did for the practice words". Participants were asked to notify the experimenter when these instructions were displayed. The experimenter then reiterated to participants that they should try to forget the words they have viewed so far. These instructions were not given in the control condition.

Stimuli. A total of 32 positive and 32 negative words (see Appendix) matched for length and frequency of use in the English language were selected from Francis and Kuçera (1982). A selection of these words had been previously used by Myers et al. (1998). 16 of the positive and 16 of the negative words were randomly selected to be rated for "self-descriptiveness", and the remaining 16 positive and negative were assigned to be rated for "other-descriptiveness". These words were presented in random order for each participant.

Distractor task. Participants counted backwards (out loud) from 200 in 3s. This lasted for approximately five minutes.

Free recall task. Control participants were asked to recall and write down on a sheet of paper, in whatever order, as many of the words they could remember rating in the task. For the experimental group they were additionally told to include all words presented, including from the list they were told to forget about. All participants were given a maximum of five minutes to complete this task.

Procedure

The study was conducted in the Cognitive Psychology Laboratory, School of Psychology, University of Leeds, in an experimental cubicle equipped with a computer with a 15 inch screen. The cubicle had a two-way mirror which had an adjustable blind fitted to it. The screen was angled so that participant and screen were facing the two-way mirror as much as possible.

Participants were brought into the lab. They were told that the experiment was investigating people's attitudes and perceptions, and that the experiment would consist of a computer task and two short questionnaires. They were advised that the experiment would take approximately 15 minutes. They then signed the consent form.

Participants in each condition were familiarised with the task in a few practice trials. After the experimenter ensured that the participant was comfortable with the task, they emphasised the instructions, private or public, respectively.

After the computer task was completed participants completed the distractor task. Then they were then given the free recall task. Finally, participants completed the STAI and the Marlowe-Crowne. After completion of the scales, participants were thanked for their cooperation. Debriefing details were given at the end of the experiment. This was to ensure that the rationale of the experiment remained anonymous until data collection ended.

RESULTS

Analyses were conducted by means of factorial analysis of variance.

Participant characteristics: Trait anxiety and defensiveness. Mean trait anxiety and defensiveness for the whole sample was 44.33 (SD = 9.83) and 13.79 (SD = 6.37), respectively. Table 1 shows the descriptive statistics for trait anxiety and defensiveness scores for participants in each of the four conditions respectively. Separate one-way ANOVAs with condition as a between-subjects factor showed that participants in the four conditions did not differ in terms of their trait anxiety scores, $F(3, 232)$ = 0.026, n.s.; and defensiveness scores, $F(3, 232)$ = 1.62, n.s.

Effects of directed forgetting instructions on words recalled. In order to see if there was a significant effect of forgetting instruction on words recalled, Univariate ANOVAs with condition (list one: forget, nonforget), as a between-

TABLE 1
Means (and standard deviations) for trait anxiety and defensiveness in the four conditions

	Private, no directed forgetting (n = 64)	*Public, no directed forgetting* (n = 56)	*Private with directed forgetting* (n = 63)	*Public with directed forgetting* (n = 53)
Trait anxiety	44.14 (9.10)	44.63 (9.90)	44.29 (10.34)	44.28 (10.26)
Defensiveness	12.50 (6.61)	15.16 (5.93)	13.98 (6.22)	13.57 (6.56)

subject factor and negative and positive words recalled as dependent variables were conducted. Analysis showed that the effect of forgetting instruction on total negative words recalled was in the predicted direction, $F(1, 233) = 3.18$, $p = .075$ (two-tailed). This finding showed that participants possessed a tendency to remember fewer negative words when instructed to forget ($M = 5.6$, $SD = 2.6$) than when not instructed to forget ($M = 6.4$, $SD = 2.9$). This showed that the experimental manipulation of forgetting instructions was on the whole successful.

Similar analysis showed no effects of forgetting instruction on positive words, $F(1, 233) = 0.001$, n.s., with participants recalling similar number of positive words in both conditions, forget ($M = 7.8$, $SD = 3.1$) and nonforget ($M = 7.9$, $SD = 3.2$). Due to no overall directed forgetting forget for positive words and the fact that there were no hypothesis for positive words the remaining experimental analyses focused exclusively on negative words.

However, we did conduct a further analysis to investigate whether the experimental manipulation was a cause for not finding a directed forgetting effect for positive words. We examined the effects of public and private manipulation on recall of positive words. Univariate ANOVAs were performed with conditions of private/public, and forget/nonforget as between-subject factors and positive words rated for self- and other- descriptiveness recalled as dependent variables. For positive self-descriptive words analysis found an interaction of private/public and forget/nonforget conditions, $F(1, 224) = 8.12$, $p = .005$. In order to follow up this interaction effect we specifically examined the effect of private and public manipulation on forgetting instructions. A Mann-Whitney test was performed for this purpose and the findings showed that forgetting instructions affected recall of positive words in the private (Mean rank = 51.13) but not public (Mean rank = 64.39) condition, $Z = -2.15$, $p = .03$.

Effects of directed forgetting instructions on the recall of to-be-forgotten words (TBF) and to-be-remembered words (TBR) as a function of private and public manipulation. Table 2 shows the descriptive statistics for negative words rated for self- and other-descriptiveness, recalled in each of the private and public conditions. Mixed ANOVA examined the effects of forgetting instructions on the recall of TBF and TBR words as a function of private and public manipulation. In this analysis condition (private forget, public forget), trait anxiety (low, high) and defensiveness (low, high) were treated as between-subject factors and list (TBF; to-be-forgotten words, TBR; to-be-remembered words) was treated as a within-subject factor, with negative words recalled rated for self-descriptiveness as the dependent variable. This analysis was performed once with trait anxiety and defensiveness median splits, and once with trait anxiety and defensiveness quartile splits. In both cases we found a significant four-way interaction of trait anxiety × defensiveness × list × condition, $F(1, 99) = 6.51$, $p = .012$ (median splits) and $F(1, 37) = 8.09$, $p = .007$ (quartile

TABLE 2
Means (and standard deviations) for negative words recalled in TBF and TBR, self or other descriptiveness, and private or public conditions for REP, LA, HA, and DHA groups using median splits

		Private		*Public*	
List		*TBF*	*TBR*	*TBF*	*TBR*
Self	REP	1.3 (0.8)	2.0 (0.8)	1.2 (0.9)	0.7 (0.7)
	LA	1.9 (0.5)	1.3 (1.0)	1.4 (1.0)	1.5 (1.1)
	HA	1.8 (1.5)	2.0 (1.0)	1.5 (1.0)	0.7 (0.8)
	DHA	1.9 (1.1)	2.1 (1.0)	0.8 (0.7)	1.2 (0.8)
Other	REP	0.8 (0.8)	1.3 (0.3)	0.7 (0.6)	0.6 (0.6)
	LA	0.8 (0.6)	1.2 (1.1)	1.1 (0.9)	1.3 (1.1)
	HA	1.1 (0.9)	1.3 (1.0)	1.1 (1.2)	0.7 (0.6)
	DHA	0.8 (0.8)	1.3 (0.4)	1.2 (1.0)	1.6 (0.5)

TBF = to-be-forgotten; TBR = to-be-remembered; REP = repressor; LA = low anxious; HA = high anxious; DHA = defensive high anxious.

splits). Both methods of analysis (i.e., using median and quartile split classification of trait anxiety and defensiveness), resulted in similar findings. This is suggestive of a strong and reliable effect of the experimental manipulations. The interaction effect (median splits) is shown in Figures 1a and 1b.

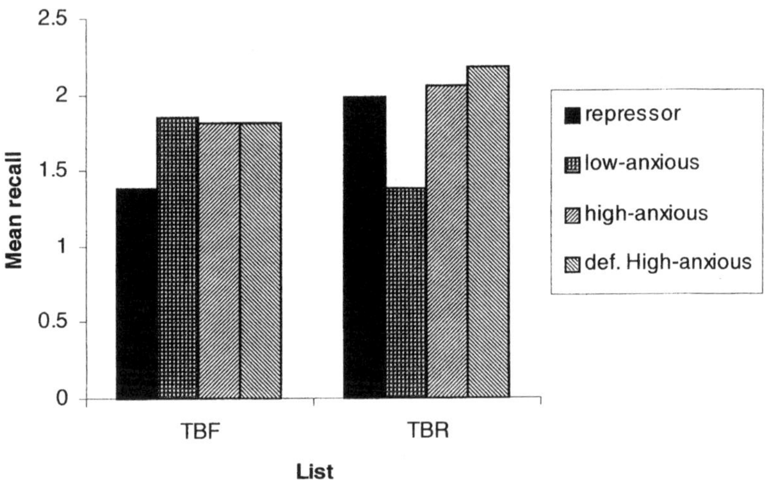

Figure 1a. Mean negative words recalled rated for self-descriptiveness from the to-be-forgotten (TBF) list and the to-be-remembered (TBR) list for the four groups in the private/forget condition.

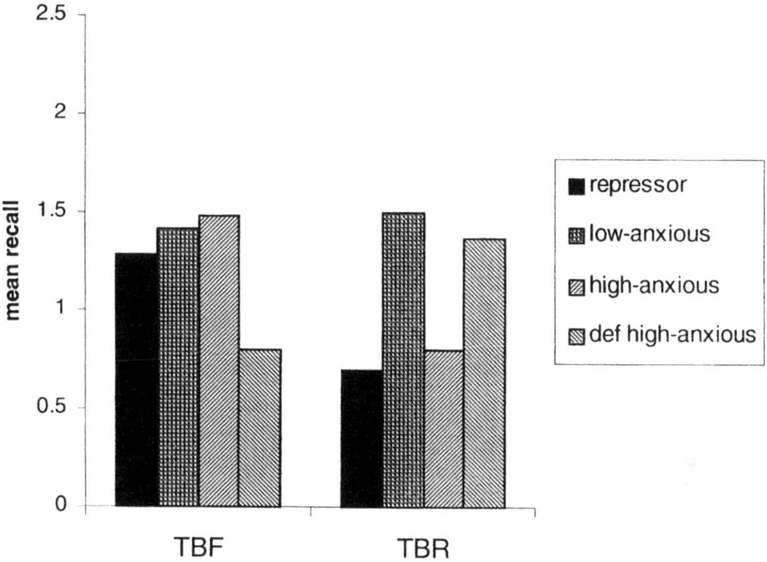

Figure 1b. Mean negative words recalled rated for self-descriptiveness from the to-be-forgotten (TBF) list and the to-be-remembered (TBR) list for the four groups in the public/forget condition.

Although the four-way interaction can be followed up and discussed in a number of possible comparisons, the focus of the experimental manipulation was on the effects of forgetting versus nonforgetting instructions. Thus it was decided to follow up the interaction effect by examining the changes between recall of TBF and TBR words for each of the repressor, low anxious, high anxious, and defensive high anxious groups in each of the private and public conditions using paired *t*-tests.

In the private condition (Figure 1a), the use of median splits on the trait anxiety and defensiveness measures resulted in 18 repressors, 11 low anxious, 21 high anxious, and 12 defensive high anxious. One-tailed paired *t*-tests showed that as predicted repressors remembered fewer TBF words than TBR words, $t(17) = -1.96$, $p = .03$. There were no significant differences between the TBF and TBR words for the low anxious, $t(10) = 1.32$, n.s., the high-anxious, $t(20) = -.42$, n.s., and defensive high anxious, $t(10) = -.58$, n.s. Similar results were obtained when quartile splits were used for repressors, $t(9) = -2.23$, $p = .026$, but given that this method resulted in very few number of participants for low anxious ($n = 3$), high anxious ($n = 8$), and defensive high anxious ($n = 4$), and hence lack of power, further results will not be discussed.

In the public condition (Figure 1b), median splits resulted in 11 repressors, 14 low anxious, 14 high anxious, and 6 defensive high anxious. One-tailed paired *t*-tests showed that the high anxious showed a significant preference for remembering more TBF than TBR words $t(13) = 2.5$, $p = .027$. There were no differences for repressors, $t(10) = 1.49$ n.s., for low anxious $t(13) = -.15$, n.s. and defensive high anxious $t(5) = -1.15$, n.s. Quartile splits resulted in very few numbers per group, low anxious ($n = 7$), repressor ($n = 3$), high anxious ($n = 5$), and defensive high anxious ($n = 5$), and thus *t*-tests were not performed.

Figures 1a and 1b show that in the private condition repressors remember significantly fewer words from the to-be-forgotten words (list 1, TBF) than the to-be-remembered words (list 2, TBR). This effect was found with both median and quartile splits on the trait anxiety and defensiveness scales, indicating a reliable effect. No other group showed a significant difference. In the public condition, the high anxious did show a significant difference with a strong tendency to remember more TBF words than TBR words.

DISCUSSION

The most striking finding of the current manipulation was that repressors forgot significantly more words in the to-be-forgotten (TBF) negative set than non-repressors, with a significant difference being found *exclusively* for self-relevant material and not for other-relevant material. This was evident only in the *private* condition and not in the public condition. To our knowledge, this study is the first to investigate the effects of forgetting as a function of private and public conditions. The findings replicate and extend Myers et al. (1998) and are consistent with the belief that repressors avoid negative information related to self (Myers, 2000). In fact, the experimental conditions in the two experiments conducted by Myers et al. (1998) could be considered equivalent to the private condition in the current study, as participants in both the Myers et al. experiments completed the directed forgetting tasks in groups of 15–20, identified by a code number to ensure anonymity. The results are also in concordance with the view that Weinberger expressed over a decade ago: "that repressors as a group, seem actively engaged in keeping themselves (rather than just other people) convinced that they are *not* prone to negative affect" (Weinberger, 1990, p. 338).

In both the current experiment and Myers et al. (1998), repressors were no worse than non-repressors at recalling the TBR negative material. In addition, in the current experiment the superior forgetting of TBF negative material by repressors was limited to the private condition, strongly highlighting that repressors' memory deficits in recalling negative material are specific rather than global.

It appears that in the private condition repressors used an avoidant strategy to inhibit negative self-relevant information but did not, or failed to effectively use this strategy, in the public condition. These results are consistent with those of Baumeister and Cairns (1992) and Derakshan and Lilja (2003). Repressors' avoidant style of processing has also been previously shown using an emotional Stroop task (e.g., Myers & McKenna, 1996; Newman & McKinney, 2002), a dichotic listening task (Bonanno, Davis, Singer, & Schwartz, 1991), a dot probe task (Fox, 1993), and an inhibition of return task (Derakshan, Feldman, Campbell, & Lipp, 2002). In fact Derakshan et al. (2002) in four experiments found that such an avoidant style of processing occurs automatically, at very early stages of processing of emotional material below the level of conscious awareness. More importantly the automatic processing style was confirmed using refined event related potential (ERP) analyses of the P3 component during early and late processing of emotional material. It seems that such inhibitory mechanisms have a physiological signature: Repressors showed enhanced P3 amplitudes, compared to nonrepressors, while performing on an attentional disengagement task. The P3 amplitude has been related to enhanced allocation of attentional resources in processing or disengaging from stimuli. Repressors also showed shorter P3 latencies, indicating a pattern of disengagement from stimuli that occurred earlier than nonrepressors. Furthermore, a recent study found that repressors compared to nonrepressors were the group most likely to avoid giving a public presentation, but were the least likely to give an emotional explanation for their avoidance (Lambie & Baker, 2003).

The fact that such forgetting of negative material was restricted to words rated for self-descriptiveness and not other-descriptiveness replicates and extends previous studies (e.g., Eysenck & Derakshan, 1997; Myers & Brewin, 1996) that the notion of threat to self-esteem in relation to avoidant strategies needs to be taken seriously. For example, Eysenck and Derakshan (1997) found that repressors rated the probability of future negative events happening to ''themselves'' as less significant than happening to ''others''. Also, repressors avoidance of self-related threat did not seem to indicate a general deficit in emotional information processing. When asked to rate levels of behavioural anxiety for self and other, repressors' minimisation of anxiety levels seemed restricted to their own behaviour, and their ratings of other's behavioural anxiety levels did not differ from independent judges' ratings (Derakshan & Eysenck, 1997). More recently, Mendolia (2002) has shown that repressive hypersensitivity and distancing of emotional material occurs only when a threat to self-concept is perceived. The current findings replicate and extend arguments that emphasise the necessity of self-relevant information in evaluating avoidant strategies employed by repressors in dealing with negative information.

The specific findings in the private condition seem to suggest a retrieval inhibition explanation of directed forgetting (see also Barnier, Levin, & Maher, this issue), rather than a deficit in encoding. It follows that if superior forgetting of self-relevant negative material was an encoding deficit there should be no differences between the private and public conditions. Caution is needed however, as there is evidence that failure to retrieve can be explained by a failure to encode emotional material (e.g., Schimmack & Hartmann, 1997). Also more recently, other explanations of the mechanisms by which directed forgetting takes place have been put forward (Sahakyan & Kelley, 2002). More research is needed to disentangle the processes involved in encoding and retrieval of emotional material (see also Shane and Peterson, this issue). For example, it would be interesting in further directed forgetting experiments to use the word method, to see whether repressors also exhibit deficits in encoding.

It is interesting that the high anxious group recalled a high number of negative words in the self-referent public TBF condition. This finding is consistent with theoretical predictions that high levels of anxiety are associated with cognitive biases, e.g. attentional biases and interpretive biases, towards threat-related and negative material (e.g., Eysenck,1992, 1997; Mathews & MacLeod, 2002; Williams, Watts, MacLeod, & Mathews, 1997). In support of this view, a previous study found that a group of high anxious individuals with obsessive compulsive disorder were poor at forgetting TBF negative words compared with positive or neutral words (Wilhelm, McNally, Baer, & Florin, 1996).

The instructions for forgetting for negative words were shown to be crucial in obtaining a directed forgetting effect for both repressors and nonrepressors. However, very surprisingly, this was not the case for positive words apart from in the self-referent private condition. To the authors' knowledge, the context in which the task has been undertaken has not been explored. Therefore, especially the private/public distinction should be further investigated in further experiments of directed forgetting.

Group differences were found with both median splits and quartile splits on anxiety and defensiveness. However, the clear results using median splits suggests that in future studies it may not be necessary to use stringent cut-offs, such as quartile splits. This would nevertheless depend in part on the nonsignificant relationship between anxiety and defensiveness. Now that is has been established that the repressor/nonrepressor difference is for the self-referent recall in the private condition, this condition can be replicated with larger numbers to investigate whether quartile splits adds anything to the findings.

The current experiment further extends the findings that repressors have a distinctive style of processing negative material related to the self, both in the laboratory tasks and when investigating their personal history. The importance of the private versus public distinction has also been highlighted. Future research should focus on the possible mechanisms that are responsible for such inhibition of threat and retrieval of such memories.

REFERENCES

Asendorpf, J. A., & Scherer, K. R. (1983). The discrepant repressor: Differentiation between low anxiety, high anxiety, and repression of anxiety by autonomic-facial-verbal patterns of behaviour. *Journal of Personality and Social Psychology*, *45*, 1334–1344.

Barnier, A. J., Levin, K., & Maher, A. (this issue). Suppressing thoughts of past events: Are repressive copers good suppressors? *Cognition and Emotion*, *18*, 513–531.

Baumeister, R. F., & Cairns, K. J. (1992). Repression and self-presentation: When audiences interfere with self-deceptive strategies. *Journal of Personality and Social Psychology*, *62*, 51–862.

Benjamins, C., Schuurs, A. H. B., & Hoogstraten, J. (1994). Skin conductance, Marlowe-Crowne, defensiveness, and dental anxiety. *Perceptual and Motor Skills*, *79*, 611–622.

Bjork, R. A. (1970). Positive forgetting: The noninterference of items intentionally forgotten. *Journal of Verbal Learning and Verbal Behaviour*, *9*, 255–268.

Bjork, R. A. (1972). Theoretical implications of directed forgetting. In A. W. Melton & E. Martin (Eds.), *Coding processes in human memory* (pp. 217–235). Washington, DC: Winston.

Boden, J. M., & Baumeister, R. F. (1997). Repressive coping: Distraction using pleasant thoughts and memories. *Journal of Personality and Social Psychology*, *73*, 1, 45–62.

Bonnano, G. A., Davis, P. J., Singer, J. L., & Schwartz, G. E. (1991). The repressor personality and avoidant information processing: A dichotic listening study. *Journal of Research in Personality*, *25*, 386–401.

Crowne, D. P., & Marlowe, D. (1964). *The approval motive: Studies in evaluative dependence.* New York: Wiley.

Davis, P. J. (1987). Repression and the inaccessibility of affective memories. *Journal of Personality and Social Psychology*, *53*, 585–593.

Davis, P. J., & Schwartz. G. E. (1987). Repression and the inaccessibility of affective memories. *Journal of Personality and Social Psychology*, *52*, 155–162.

Derakshan, N., & Eysenck, M. W. (1997). Interpretive biases for one's own behaviour and physiology in high trait-anxious individuals and repressors. *Journal of Personality and Social Psychology*, *73*, 816–825.

Derakshan, N., & Eysenck, M. W. (1998). Working memory capacity in high trait-anxious and repressor groups. *Cognition and Emotion*, *12*, 697–713.

Derakshan, N., & Eysenck, M. W. (1999). Are repressors self-deceivers or other-deceivers? *Cognition & Emotion*, *13*, 1–17.

Derakshan, N., & Eysenck, M. W. (2001a). Manipulation of focus of attention and its effects on anxiety in high-anxious individuals and repressors. *Anxiety, Stress, and Coping*, *14*, 173–191.

Derakshan, N., & Eysenck, M. W. (2001b). Effects of focus of attention on physiological, behavioural, and self-reported anxiety in high-anxious, low-anxious, defensive high-anxious, and repressors. *Anxiety, Stress, and Coping*, *14*, 285–299.

Derakshan, N., & Lilja, N. (2003). *Self-deception and other-deception: Two sides of the same coin?* Unpublished manuscript.

Derakshan, N., Feldman, M., Campbell, T., & Lipp, O. (2002). Don't look back to emotion: Inhibited to return to emotion: Investigating the time course of attentional bias. *Psychophysiology*, *39*, S31.

Eysenck, M. W. (1992). *Anxiety: The cognitive perspective.* Hove, UK: Lawrence Erlbaum Associates Ltd.

Eysenck, M. W. (1997). *Anxiety and cognition: A unified theory.* Hove, UK: Psychology Press.

Eysenck, M. W., & Derakshan, N. (1997). Cognitive biases for future negative events as a function of trait anxiety and social desirability. *Personality and Individual Differences*, *22*, 597–605.

Fox, E. (1993). Allocation of visual attention and anxiety. *Cognition and Emotion*, *7*, 207–215.

Francis, W. N., & Kuçera, H. (1982). *Frequency analysis of English usage.* Boston: Houghton Miffin.

Geiselman, R. E., Bjork, R. A., & Fishman, D. L. (1983). Disrupted retrieval in directed forgetting: A link with posthypnotic amnesia. *Journal of Experimental Psychology: General*, *112*, 58–72.

Jensen, M. R. (1987). Psychobiological factors predicting the course of breast cancer. *Journal of Personality*, *55*, 317–342.

Jongeward, R. H., Woodward A. E., & Bjork, R. A. (1975). The relative roles of input and output mechanisms in directed forgetting. *Memory and Cognition*, *3*, 51–57.

Korfine, L., & Hooley, J. M. (2000). Directed forgetting of emotional stimuli in borderline personality disorder. *Journal of Abnormal Psychology*, *109*, 214–221.

Lambie, J. A., & Baker, K. L. (2003). Intentional avoidance and social understanding in repressors and non-repressors: Two functions of emotional experience? *Consciousness and Emotion*, *26*, 17–42.

Mathews, A., & MacLeod, C. (2002). Induced processing biases have causal effects on anxiety. *Cognition and Emotion, 16*, 331–353.

McNally, R. J., Clancy, S. A., Barrett, H. M., & Parker, H. A. (this issue). Inhibiting retrieval of trauma cues in adults reporting histories of childhood sexual abuse. *Cognition and Emotion, 18*, 479–493.

Mendolia, M. (2002). An index of self-regulation of emotion and the study of repression in social contexts that threaten or do not threaten self-concepts. *Emotion, 2*, 215–232.

Moulds, M. L., & Bryant, R. A. (2002). Directed forgetting in acute stress disorder. *Journal of Abnormal Psychology, 111*, 175–179.

Myers, L. B. (2000). Identifying repressors: A methodological issue for health psychology. *Psychology and Health, 15*, 205–214.

Myers, L. B., & Brewin, C. R. (1994). Recall of early experience and the repressive coping style. *Journal of Abnormal Psychology, 103*, 288–292.

Myers, L. B., & Brewin, C. R. (1995). Repressive coping and the recall of emotional material. *Cognition and Emotion, 9*, 637–642.

Myers, L. B., & Brewin, C. R. (1996). illusions of well-being and the repressive coping style. *British Journal of Social Psychology, 33*, 443–457.

Myers, L. B., Brewin, C. R., & Power, M. J. (1998). Repressive coping and the directed forgetting of emotional material. *Journal of Abnormal Psychology, 107*, 141–148.

Myers, L. B., Brewin, C. R., & Power, M. J. (1992). Repression and autobiographical memory. In M. A. Conway, D. C. Rubin, H. Spinnler, and W. Wagenaar (Eds.), *Theoretical perspectives on autobiographical memory* (pp. 375–390). Dordrecht: Kluwer.

Myers, L. B., & McKenna, F. P. (1996). The colour naming of socially threatening words. *Personality and Individual Differences, 6*, 801–803.

Newman, L. S., & McKinney, L. C. (2002). Repressive coping and threat avoidance: An idiographic Stroop Study. *Personality and Social Psychology Bulletin, 28*, 409–422.

Newton, T. L., & Contrada, R. L. (1992). Repressive coping and verbal-autonomic dissociation: The influence of social context. *Journal of Personality and Social Psychology, 62*, 159–167.

Niaura, R., Herbert. P. N., McMahon, N., & Sommerville, L. (1992). Repressive coping and blood lipids in men and women. *Psychosomatic Medicine, 54*, 698–706.

Power, M. J., Dalgleish, T., Claudio, V., Tata, P., & Kentish, J. (2000). The directed forgetting task: application to emotionally valent material. *Journal of affective disorders, 57*, 147–157.

Sahakyan, L., & Kelley, C. M. (2002). A contextual change account of the directed forgetting effect. *Journal of Experimental Psychology. Learning, Memory, and Cognition, 28*, 1064–1072.

Schimmack, U., & Hartmann, K. (1997). Individual differences in the memory representation of emotional episodes: exploring the cognitive processes in repression. *Journal of Personality and Social Psychology, 73*, 1064–1079.

Shane, M. S., & Peterson, J. B. (this issue). Self-induced distortions and the allocation of processing resources at encoding and retrieval. *Cognition and Emotion, 18*, 533–558.

Spielberger, C. D., Gorsuch, R. L., Lushene, R., Vagg, P. R., & Jacobs, G. A. (1983). *Manual for the state-trait anxiety inventory*. Palo Alto, CA: Consulting Psychologists Press.

Tolin, D. F., Hamlin, C., & Foa, E. (2002). Directed forgetting in obsessive compulsive disorder: Replication and extension. *Behaviour Research and Therapy, 40*, 792–803.

Weinberger, D. A. (1990). The construct validity of the repressive coping style. In J. L. Singer (Ed.), *Repression and dissociation* (pp. 337–386). Chicago: University of Chicago Press.

Weinberger, D. A., Schwartz, G. E., & Davidson, J. R. (1979). Low-anxious, high-anxious, and repressive coping styles: Psychometric patterns and behavioural and physiological responses to stress. *Journal of Abnormal Psychology, 88*, 369–380.

Wilhelm, S., McNally, R. J., Baer, L., & Florin, I. (1996). Directed forgetting in obsessive-compulsive disorder. *Behaviour, Research and Therapy, 34*, 633–641.

Williams, J. M. G., Watts, F. N., MacLeod, C., Mathews, A. (1997). *Cognitive psychology and emotional disorders* (2nd ed.). Chichester: Wiley.

APPENDIX

Words used in the directed forgetting task

Negative words	*Positive words*
risky	merry
jumpy	helpful
worried	honourable
anxious	relaxed
suspicious	exuberant
frightened	sociable
fearful	praiseworthy
furious	resourceful
horrified	respectful
disgusted	patient
outraged	jolly
grieving	excited
unattractive	productive
unreasonable	amusing
thoughtless	fulfilled
pessimistic	ecstatic
despondent	entertaining
irrational	considerate
selfish	purposeful
unhappy	sincere
guilty	eager
lonely	enthusiastic
ugly	generous
rejected	confident
nervous	ambitious
useless	brave
defensive	lively
inadequate	delightful
stupid	peaceful
troubled	relieved
mean	charming
lucky	aggressive

COGNITION AND EMOTION, 2004, *18* (4), 513–531

Suppressing thoughts of past events: Are repressive copers good suppressors?

Amanda J. Barnier, Kirsty Levin, and Alena Maher
University of New South Wales, Sydney, Australia

We investigated the ability of individuals with a "repressive coping style" to strategically control thoughts of events from their past, which made them feel either proud or embarrassed, within the thought suppression paradigm. We examined whether (low) anxiety and (high) defensiveness interacts to influence suppression success over and above anxiety and defensiveness alone using low anxious, repressor, high anxious, and defensive high anxious groups. For the emotionally positive "proud event", all groups avoided event-related thoughts when instructed to suppress. For the emotionally negative "embarrassed event", repressors reported fewer event-related thoughts than all other groups, even when not instructed to suppress. Repressors also reported the lowest level of suppression effort and showed no "rebound". We discuss repressors' memory performance in terms of their natural tendency to avoid negative self-referent material, and thought and memory control in everyday life.

There is increasing evidence that in everyday life individuals may use inhibitory processing strategies to regulate their awareness of memories and thoughts they find threatening or painful (Bjork, Bjork, & Anderson, 1998; Dalgleish, Mathews, & Wood, 1999; Koutstaal & Schacter, 1997). Bjork (1989) defined retrieval inhibition as "a suppression-type process directed at the to-be-inhibited information for some adaptive purpose" (p. 324), which results in the loss of retrieval access to, but not availability of, certain memory material. Clinical disorders, such as functional amnesia, posttraumatic stress disorder, dissociative fugue, and dissociative identity disorder, offer extreme examples of the inhibition or avoidance of personal memories (Brewin, 2001; Kihlstrom & Schacter,

---

Correspondence should be addressed to Amanda J. Barnier, School of Psychology, University of New South Wales, Sydney NSW 2052, Australia; e-mail: A.Barnier@unsw.edu.au

This research was supported by a Queen Elizabeth II Fellowship and Large Grant from the Australian Research Council and a University Research Support Program Grant from the University of New South Wales to Amanda Barnier. We are grateful for that support. We are grateful also to Rochelle Cox and Lissa Johnson for research assistance, and to Daniel B. Wright and an anonymous reviewer for their comments on an earlier draft of this manuscript.

http://www.tandf.co.uk/journals/pp/02699931.html DOI:10.1080/02699930341000428

1995).[1] Although there has been significant debate about the precise mechanism underlying self-initiated memory management (McNally, 2003), the notion that individuals protect themselves by avoiding negative material is consistent with goal-directed models of autobiographical memory (Conway & Pleydell-Pearce, 2000; McAdams, 2001; Singer & Salovey, 1993).

There is evidence also that some individuals are particularly adept at using these protective processing strategies. Weinberger (1990; see also Eysenck, 2000) identified individuals with a "repressive coping style", who score low on self-report measures of trait anxiety but high on self-report measures of defensiveness; he contrasted "repressive copers" (or "repressors") with low anxious (low anxiety, low defensiveness), high anxious (high anxiety, low defensiveness), and defensive high anxious (high anxiety, high defensiveness) individuals. Repressors are highly physiologically reactive in potentially stressful situations, yet report low levels of distress (e.g., Derakshan & Eysenck, 1997, 2001; Weinberger, Schwartz, & Davidson, 1979). Also, they demonstrate an avoidant attentional style (e.g., Bonnano, Davis, Singer, & Schwartz, 1991; Newman & McKinney, 2002). Weinberger (1990) argued that "repressors fail to recognize their own affective responses ... [and] are likely to employ a variety of strategies to avoid conscious knowledge of their 'genuine reactions' " (p. 338).

One important and consistent finding is that repressors' defensive style leads to characteristic memory deficits. Repressors have difficulty recalling negatively valenced information, both when the material is personally generated (e.g., autobiographical memories in a cued recall task) and when it is experimentally generated (e.g., lists of words in a directed forgetting task). For instance, Davis (1987; see also Davis, 1990; Davis & Schwartz, 1987; Myers & Brewin, 1994; Newman & Hedberg, 1999) asked repressors and nonrepressors to generate autobiographical memories from childhood in response to positive and negative emotional cue words (e.g., happy, angry).[2] Whereas repressors recalled a similar number of positive memories to nonrepressors, they recalled fewer negative memories; when they managed to recall negative memories, their recall latencies were much longer. Within a list-method directed forgetting procedure, Myers, Brewin, and Power (1998) asked repressors and nonrepressors to rate two sets of positive and negative adjectives in terms of self-descriptiveness (i.e., how

[1] Inhibition can be understood on at least three levels: as lowering the expression of memory at recall (i.e., the behavioural level), as lowering the accessibility of memory (i.e., the retrieval level), and as lowering the activation of the memory representation itself (i.e., the accessibility level). The behavioural level entails the weakest, descriptive sense of inhibition, whereas the accessibility level entails the strongest, mechanistic sense. In this research, we conceptualise inhibition in terms of the expression and accessibility of memory (for discussion of the concept of inhibition, see Anderson, Bjork, & Bjork, 1994; Dalgleish et al., 1999).

[2] In this literature, nonrepressor comparison groups typically involve a combined group of low anxious, high anxious, defensive high anxious, and/or nonextreme scoring individuals.

descriptive they were of themselves). They told participants that the first set of words were unimportant and could be forgotten and to focus on the second set of words. Whereas both repressors and nonrepressors later recalled fewer words from the first than the second set (i.e., a directed forgetting effect; Bjork, 1989), only repressors were influenced by the emotional valence of the words; they recalled fewer negative self-descriptive words from the first, to-be-forgotten, set than nonrepressors.

These data suggest that repressors are not only better able or more likely to use inhibitory processing strategies, but that their use of these strategies is selective. Davis (1990) argued that repressors' use of inhibitory strategies ''may be motivated in particular by affective experiences that focus attention on the self in a threatening or evaluative way'' (p. 585). Research confirms that only negative self-referent information engages the repressive coping style (e.g., self-descriptive not other-descriptive negative adjectives; Barnier, 2001). In other words, individuals with a repressive coping style may be good ''repressors'' in Freud's (1915/1957; see also Erdelyi, 1990) sense—they selectively and successfully avoid negative information that threatens the self.

Although previous research highlights the nature of the material that engages repressors' use of inhibitory processes or strategies, it is less clear whether these processes represent: (a) an automatic response to particular information; (b) strategic, motivated attempts to control awareness of certain memories; or (c) a combination of these (Dalgleish et al., 1999). Procedures such as cued autobiographical recall and directed forgetting do not allow clear predictions that differentiate between these possible mechanisms to be made. To address this issue we examined repressors' management of negative self-referent material within Wegner's (1994) thought suppression paradigm. This procedure focuses on individuals' ability to successfully avoid or control conscious (and in some cases unwanted and intrusive) thoughts, images, memories or feelings about a topic. In their classic experiment, Wegner, Schneider, Carter, and White (1987, experiment 1) asked participants to try not to think of a white bear and collected continuous stream-of-consciousness reports following the instruction. Although participants showed some initial success in suppressing thoughts of the white bear during this suppression period, the instruction lead to a ''rebound effect'' whereby they thought of the bear during a subsequent expression period more often than those who had not been asked to suppress. Wegner's (1994; Wenzlaff & Wegner, 2000) theory of ironic processes explains these findings in terms of two mechanisms: an intentional operating process that seeks thoughts that will promote successful suppression of the unwanted thought; and an ironic monitoring process that remains in the background of consciousness and searches for mental contents that indicate a failure to suppress the unwanted thought. Laying aside this interpretation, the thought suppression procedure allows us to compare repressors' ''strategic'' (suppression instruction) versus ''natural'' (no instruction) levels of suppression.

To maximise the chance of engaging individuals' repressive coping style, and to link more obviously with both everyday thought control and clinical disorders of memory (Koutstaal & Schacter, 1997; Rassin, Merckelbach, & Muris, 2000), we asked repressors and nonrepressors to recall a recent event during which they felt extremely proud (''proud event'') and an event during which they felt extremely embarrassed (''embarrassed event''). These emotional self-relevant autobiographical memories became the target for suppression. This is important because both emotional and self-relevant material show different outcomes within the thought suppression paradigm to neutral, nonpersonal material (Wenzlaff & Wegner, 2000). For instance, McNally and Ricciardi (1996) found that whereas reports of a neutral thought (white bear) decreased from the suppression to expression periods, reports of a negative personally relevant thought increased threefold. When other variables are equal, emotional (particularly negative) material may be more difficult to suppress than neutral material (see also Howell & Conway, 1992; Markowitz & Borton, 2002; for a review, see Wenzlaff & Wegner, 2000). However, we expected that repressors would be good, ''natural'' suppressors, especially of negative self-referent material.

Rather than comparing repressors simply with a combined group of nonrepressors, we used four groups of participants based on Weinberger et al.'s (1979) fourfold classification scheme: low anxious, repressor, high anxious, and defensive high anxious individuals. This allows us to examine whether the interaction of anxiety and defensiveness (i.e., the repressive coping style) influences suppression success over and above anxiety and defensiveness alone. Our thought suppression procedure involved three experimental periods. In an *imaging period*, participants generated and focused on a recent proud event or a recent embarrassed event. In a *suppression period*, participants were instructed either to avoid all thoughts of the target event (*suppression condition*) or to think of anything (*nonsuppression condition*); all participants monitored thought intrusions by pressing a button each time an event-related thought came to mind. In an *expression period*, all participants were invited to think of anything and again monitored event-related thoughts. Participants completed this sequence of imaging, suppression, and expression first for their proud event and then for their embarrassed event, or first for their embarrassed event and then for their proud event.

Based on findings of repressors' memory biases and findings of thought suppression for emotional material, we expected an interaction between anxiety and defensiveness for the embarrassed event but not for the proud event. Specifically, for the proud event, we expected that all participants instructed to suppress would report fewer thought intrusions than those not instructed to suppress. However, for the embarrassed event, we expected that thought suppression would be more successful and less effortful for repressors than for all other groups, irrespective of instruction. The thought suppression paradigm also predicts postsuppression rebound following a period of successful suppression (although its degree depends on the nature of the targeted material; for reviews, see Abramowitz, Tolin, & Street, 2001; Renaud & McConnell, 2002). We expected that repressors would be skilled at avoiding this phenomenon and would not show rebound (particularly of their embarrassed event) irrespective of an instruction to suppress and initial suppression success.

METHOD

Participants and design

A total of 84 (28 male, 56 female) undergraduate psychology students from the University of New South Wales, Sydney, Australia were tested in a 2 (anxiety: low vs. high) × 2 (defensiveness: low vs. high) × 2 (instruction: suppression vs. nonsuppression) × (2) (event: proud vs. embarrassed) mixed-model design. They participated in return for credit towards their psychology course, and ranged in age from 17 to 44 years (M = 19.04, SD = 3.34).

Consistent with participant selection in previous studies (e.g., Derakshan & Eysenck, 1999, 2001; Myers et al., 1998; Vetere & Myers, 2002), students were identified and categorised as low anxious (low anxiety, low defensiveness), repressor (low anxiety, high defensiveness), high anxious (high anxiety, low defensiveness), and defensive high anxious (high anxiety, high defensiveness) based on their scores on measures of anxiety (Spielberger Stait-Trait Anxiety Inventory [STAI]: Spielberger, Gorsuch, Lushene, Vagg, & Jacobs, 1983; range 20–80) and defensiveness (MC: Crowne & Marlowe, 1964; range 0–33). Based on third-splits, low anxiety was defined as a STAI score $\leq$ 39 and high anxiety was a STAI score $\geq$ 49. Low defensiveness was defined as a MC score $\leq$ 12 and high defensiveness was a MC score $\geq$ 17.

Selected from a larger pool of 260 respondents, the sample included: 24 low anxious (9 male, 15 female) with low STAI (M = 34.96, SD = 3.13) and low MC (M = 9.50, SD = 2.65) scores; 24 repressor (5 male, 19 female) with low STAI (M = 31.33, SD = 4.92) and high MC (M = 21.33, SD = 2.53) scores; 24 high anxious (11 male, 13 female) with high STAI (M = 54.00, SD = 7.02) and low MC (M = 8.71, SD = 2.93) scores; and 12 defensive high anxious (3 male, 9 female) with high STAI (M = 54.92, SD = 4.80) and high MC (M = 19.58, SD = 1.51) scores.[3]

Materials and apparatus

Participants' event-related thoughts during the suppression and expression periods were recorded using a joystick button connected to a DOS-based computer program, which recorded the frequency of button presses in 500

[3] The smaller number of defensive high anxious participants reflects the fact that the combination of extremely high levels of both anxiety and defensiveness is less common in screening samples than other profiles (Weinberger et al., 1979).

millisecond increments. The joystick was placed on the left arm of participants' chair. Configuration and activation of the program was controlled by the experimenter via a keyboard. For each (proud or embarrassed) autobiographical event, the program recorded for a total of 6 minutes across the suppression and expression periods.

Procedure

The experiment involved two experimental phases corresponding to the two autobiographical events. Each experimental phase consisted of imaging, suppression, and expression periods interspersed with sets of subjective ratings. The two experimental phases were structurally and procedurally identical except that half the participants focused first on an event that made them feel proud followed by an event that made them feel embarrassed, and half focused first on their embarrassed event followed by their proud event. Initial analyses indicated that order of event elicitation had no impact on performance, so the two event orders were collapsed in the analyses reported below. A mathematical filler task separated the experimental phases. Participants were tested in individual sessions and sat in an armchair facing the experimenter.

Imaging period. To begin, the experimenter told participants that they were taking part in an experiment examining the persistence of thoughts in everyday life and their task was to recall and think about two autobiographical events from their past. She asked participants to think of a memory of a specific event they had experienced in the last 12 months; she asked half to think of an event during which they felt extremely proud, and half to think of an event during which they felt extremely embarrassed. She then asked for a brief general description of the remembered event; to minimise self-editing, the experimenter emphasised that there was no need to reveal private or confidential details of the memories. Following this, the experimenter asked participants to close their eyes and to think further about their remembered event. She asked them to think back and to focus on exactly what happened, who was involved, and how they felt. After 2 minutes, the experimenter asked participants to open their eyes and to rate the valence (1 = *very negative*, 10 = *very positive*) and clarity/vividness (1 = *not at all clear/vivid*, 10 = *very clear/vivid*) of their memory, as well as how anxious (1 = *not at all anxious*, 10 = *extremely anxious*) and distressed (1 = *not at all distressed*, 10 = *very distressed*) they felt while thinking of the event.

Suppression period. The experimenter gave participants a computer joystick with a button on top and said that for the next 2 minutes they should use the button to monitor their thoughts. She then administered either suppression or nonsuppression instructions; there were two versions of the suppression instruction. She gave one third of participants an instruction to suppress the entire event ("I want you to not think about the event during which you felt extremely proud/embarrassed. You can think about anything else, but do not think about that event or anything to do with it"), one third an instruction to suppress the emotional aspects of the event ("I want you to not think about the event during which you felt extremely proud/embarrassed; in particular, I want you to not think about the feelings involved"), and one third nonsuppression instructions ("I want you to think about anything. You might think about the event during which you felt extremely proud/embarrassed or you might not."). Initial analyses indicated that the wording of the suppression instruction had no impact on performance, so the two versions were collapsed into one condition (16 low anxious, 16 repressor, 16 high anxious, 8 defensive high anxious) and compared with the nonsuppression condition (8 low anxious, 8 repressor, 8 high anxious, 4 defensive high anxious).

The experimenter asked all participants to monitor the content of their thoughts and to press the joystick button each time they had a thought related to their remembered event. She encouraged them to honestly report all event-related thoughts. Participants closed their eyes and monitored their thoughts until the experimenter indicated that 2 minutes had elapsed. Following this, the experimenter asked participants to open their eyes and to rate how often they thought about the event during this period (frequency: 1 = *not at all*, 10 = *all the time*), how hard they tried not to think about the event (effort: 1 = *not at all hard*, 10 = *very hard*), and how successful they thought they were in suppressing event-related thoughts (success: 1 = *not at all successful*, 10 = *very successful*).

Expression period. The experimenter asked participants to focus again on the joystick and said that for the next 2 minutes they should use the button to again monitor their thoughts. She told all participants that they could "spend the next two minutes thinking about anything you like. You might like to think about the event during which you felt extremely proud/embarrassed or you might not". She asked them to honestly monitor the content of their thoughts in the same way as during the suppression period. Participants closed their eyes and monitored their thoughts until the experimenter indicated that 2 minutes had elapsed. Following this, the experimenter asked participants to open their eyes and to make the same ratings of intrusion frequency, suppression effort, and suppression success as during the suppression period.

This was the end of the first experimental phase. The experimenter asked participants to complete a 5 minute mathematical filler task while she reset the joystick program and then began the second phase. This phase was identical to the first phase with the exception that participants who were initially asked to focus on an event during which they felt extremely proud, now focused on an event during which they felt extremely embarrassed, and participants who focused on their embarrassed event, now focused on their proud event. At the end of the second experimental phase, participants were invited to ask questions, debriefed, and thanked for their time.

RESULTS

Autobiographical events selected during the imaging period

All 84 participants generated memories of events that made them feel proud and embarrassed as requested. These memories differed in terms of emotional significance and quality. A 2 (anxiety) × 2 (defensiveness) × 2 (instruction) × (2) ANOVA of participants' ratings of emotional valence yielded a main effect of event, $F(1, 76) = 233.10$, $p < .001$, $\eta_p^2 = .754$, and an interaction between event and defensiveness, $F(1, 76) = 4.51$, $p = .037$, $\eta_p^2 = .056$.[4] Participants rated their proud events as very positive ($M = 8.29$, $SD = 1.41$) and their embarrassed events as quite negative ($M = 4.31$, $SD = 1.78$). High defensive individuals (repressor and defensive high anxious) rated their embarrassed event as slightly more negative ($M = 3.92$, $SD = 1.61$) than low defensive individuals (low anxious and high anxious; $M = 4.60$, $SD = 1.85$); there was no difference for their proud event. A similar 2 × 2 × 2 × (2) ANOVA of ratings of clarity/vividness yielded an interaction between event and anxiety, $F(1, 76) = 4.17$, $p = .045$, $\eta_p^2 = .052$. Overall, participants rated their memories of the proud ($M = 8.37$, $SD = 1.53$) and embarrassed ($M = 7.88$, $SD = 1.72$) events as very clear and vivid. However, whereas high anxiety individuals (high anxious and defensive high anxious) rated their proud ($M = 8.06$, $SD = 1.71$) and embarrassed ($M = 8.08$, $SD = 1.73$) events similarly, low anxiety individuals (low anxious and repressor) rated their embarrassed event ($M = 7.73$, $SD = 1.72$) as slightly less clear than their proud event ($M = 8.60$, $SD = 1.35$).

A 2 (anxiety) × 2 (defensiveness) × 2 (instruction) × (2) (event) mixed-model ANOVA of participants' ratings of anxiety during the imaging period yielded main effects of event and anxiety, $F(1, 76) = 4.62$, $p = .035$, $\eta_p^2 = .057$ and $F(1, 76) = 3.95$, $p = .050$, $\eta_p^2 = .049$, respectively, and an interaction between anxiety and defensiveness, $F(1, 76) = 4.42$, $p = .039$, $\eta_p^2 = .055$. A similar 2 × 2 × 2 × (2) ANOVA of ratings of distress during this period also yielded main effects of event and anxiety, $F(1, 76) = 35.29$, $p < .001$, $\eta_p^2 = .317$ and $F(1, 76) = 4.84$, $p = .031$, $\eta_p^2 = .060$, respectively; and interactions between event and anxiety and between anxiety and defensiveness, $F(1, 76) = 4.54$, $p = .036$, $\eta_p^2 = .056$ and $F(1, 76) = 4.63$, $p = .035$, $\eta_p^2 = .057$, respectively. Participants felt more anxious and distressed while thinking about their embarrassed event (anxiety: $M = 3.81$, $SD = 2.47$; distress: $M = 3.01$, $SD = 2.29$) than their

[4] Partial eta squared (η_p^2) was used to estimate the strength of association for each effect in ANOVA. Tabachnick and Fidell (1996) recommended its use because, unlike eta squared (η^2), it is not influenced by the number and significance of other independent variables in the design.

proud event (anxiety: $M = 3.21$, $SD = 2.13$; distress: $M = 1.60$, $SD = 1.11$). Also, high anxiety individuals (high anxious and defensive high anxious; anxiety: $M = 3.79$, $SD = 1.56$; distress: $M = 2.58$, $SD = 1.45$) reported more anxiety and distress than low anxiety individuals (low anxious and repressor; anxiety: $M = 3.30$, $SD = 1.79$; distress: $M = 2.09$, $SD = 1.29$). Finally, repressors reported lower levels of anxiety ($M = 3.10$, $SD = 1.84$) and distress ($M = 1.88$, $SD = 1.24$) than low anxious (anxiety: $M = 3.50$, $SD = 1.77$; distress: $M = 2.31$, $SD = 2.31$), high anxious (anxiety: $M = 3.46$, $SD = 1.39$; distress: $M = 2.46$, $SD = 1.37$), and defensive high anxious (anxiety: $M = 4.46$, $SD = 3.79$; distress: $M = 2.83$, $SD = 1.64$) individuals.

In summary, participants generated appropriate positive (proud) and negative (embarrassed) memories as targets for suppression. The proud and embarrassed events differed in valence, but not vividness and clarity. Whereas all participants (particularly high anxiety individuals) felt more anxious and distressed when thinking about their embarrassed event, repressors reported the lowest levels of negative affect.

Suppression success

Table 1 presents participants' mean number of event-related thoughts (as indicated by button presses) during the suppression period for the proud and embarrassed events. To index the distribution of these thoughts across groups, instructions, and events, Table 2 presents minimum, maximum, median, and mode values. A 2 (anxiety) × 2 (defensiveness) × 2 (instruction) × (2) (event) mixed-model ANOVA of this data yielded main effects of anxiety, $F(1, 76) = 7.47$, $p = .008$, $\eta_p^2 = .090$, defensiveness, $F(1, 76) = 3.46$, $p = .067$, $\eta_p^2 = .043$, and instruction, $F(1, 76) = 13.22$, $p = .001$, $\eta_p^2 = .148$. It also yielded a near significant interaction between anxiety and instruction, $F(1, 76) = 3.46$, $p = .067$, $\eta_p^2 = .043$. To test the prediction that repressors would show characteristic avoidance of their embarrassed event irrespective of suppression instruction, we conducted follow-up 2 (anxiety) × 2 (defensiveness) × 2 (instruction) ANOVAs for the proud and embarrassed events separately.

For the proud event, the follow-up ANOVA yielded only main effects of anxiety (near significant) and instruction, $F(1, 76) = 3.59$, $p = .062$, $\eta_p^2 = .045$ and $F(1, 76) = 9.77$, $p = .003$, $\eta_p^2 = .114$, respectively. As expected within the thought suppression paradigm, individuals told to suppress ($M = 3.05$, $SD = 2.25$) reported fewer event-related thoughts than individuals not told to suppress ($M = 4.82$, $SD = 3.36$). Also, low anxiety individuals (low anxious and repressor; $M = 3.19$, $SD = 2.32$) reported fewer event-related thoughts than high anxiety individuals (high anxious and defensive high anxious; $M = 4.25$, $SD = 3.23$). Overall, all participants suppressed thoughts of their proud event when instructed.

TABLE 1
Mean number (and standard deviations) of event-related thoughts during the suppression period

Anxiety and defensiveness	*Instruction*	
	Suppression	*Nonsuppression*
Proud event		
Low anxiety		
Low defensiveness (LA)	3.63 (2.36)	4.00 (3.16)
High defensiveness (REP)	1.88 (1.36)	4.13 (2.03)
High anxiety		
Low defensiveness (HA)	3.81 (2.59)	5.63 (5.01)
High defensiveness (DHA)	2.75 (2.05)	6.25 (1.50)
Embarrassed event		
Low anxiety		
Low defensiveness (LA)	3.75 (3.70)	4.75 (4.06)
High defensiveness (REP)	1.69 (1.40)	2.13 (1.55)
High anxiety		
Low defensiveness (HA)	3.50 (2.88)	7.38 (6.09)
High defensiveness (DHA)	2.88 (1.13)	6.25 (3.86)

Note: LA = low anxious; REP = repressor; HA = high anxious; DHA = defensive high anxious.

For the embarrassed event, the follow-up ANOVA yielded main effects of anxiety, $F(1, 76) = 6.03$, $p = .016$, $\eta_p^2 = .074$, defensiveness, $F(1, 76) = 4.23$, $p = .043$, $\eta_p^2 = .053$, and instruction, $F(1, 76) = 7.70$, $p = .007$, $\eta_p^2 = .092$. It also yielded a near significant interaction between anxiety and instruction, $F(1, 76) = 3.45$, $p = .067$, $\eta_p^2 = .043$. Again, as expected within this paradigm, individuals told to suppress (M = 2.96, SD = 3.04) reported fewer event-related thoughts than individuals not told to suppress (M = 4.53, SD = 3.94). Also, whereas low anxiety individuals (low anxious and repressor; M = 2.96, SD = 3.04) reported fewer event-related thoughts than high anxiety individuals (high anxious and defensive high anxious; M = 4.53, SD = 3.94), low defensive individuals (low anxious and high anxious; M = 4.44, SD = 4.09) reported more event-related thoughts than high defensive individuals (repressor and defensive high anxious; M = 2.56, SD = 2.20).

Although there was no statistical interaction between anxiety and defensiveness, inspection of Table 1 reveals that, numerically at least, repressors reported fewer event-related thoughts of their embarrassed event than all other groups in both the suppression and nonsuppression conditions. The distribution data in Table 2 suggests that repressors' mean number of reported thoughts was not an artifact of a few participants. Rather, there was little variance in their thought suppression performance for the embarrassed event; the range of

TABLE 2
Range, median, and mode of event-related thoughts during the suppression period

	Instruction					
	Suppression			*Nonsuppression*		
Anxiety and defensiveness	*Range*	*Median*	*Mode*	*Range*	*Median*	*Mode*
Proud event						
Low anxiety						
Low defensiveness (LA)	0–7	3.5	2,6	0–10	3.5	2,4
High defensiveness (REP)	0–5	2	2	1–7	4.5	5
High anxiety						
Low defensiveness (HA)	1–10	3	1,2,3	1–16	4	1,4
High defensiveness (DHA)	0–6	2	2	5–8	6	5
Embarrassed event						
Low anxiety						
Low defensiveness (LA)	0–15	3	3	0–13	4	4
High defensiveness (REP)	0–5	1	1	0–4	2	1
High anxiety						
Low defensiveness (HA)	0–8	3	1	0–18	7.5	none
High defensiveness (DHA)	1–4	3	4	2–10	6.5	2,4,9,10

Note: LA, low anxious; REP = repressor; HA = high anxious; DHA = defensive high anxious. For some groups there was more than one mode. There was no mode for HA individuals in nonsuppression (embarrassed event); reported thoughts for these eight participants were 0, 1, 3, 6, 9, 10, 12, and 18.

reported thoughts was only 0 to 4 or 5, and the median and mode were very low at 1 or 2. This is particularly notable in the nonsuppression condition, where repressors' thoughts of the embarrassed event ranged from 0 to 4 in comparison to 0–13 for low anxious, 0–18 for high anxious, and 2–10 for defensive high anxious individuals. In other words, only repressors consistently suppressed thoughts of their embarrassed event irrespective of suppression instruction.

Subjective effort and success of suppression

Participants' ratings of thought frequency were strongly correlated with the number of reported thoughts as indicated by button presses (proud event: $r = .64$, $p < .001$; embarrassed event: $r = .62$, $p < .001$). Participants also rated their suppression effort and suppression success. A 2 (anxiety) × 2 (defensiveness) × 2 (instruction) × (2) (event) mixed-model ANOVA of participants' ratings of effort yielded main effects of anxiety (near-significant) and instruction, $F(1, 76) = 3.34$, $p = .072$, $\eta_p^2 = .042$ and $F(1, 76) = 7.69$, $p = .007$, $\eta_p^2 = .092$, respectively. It also yielded a near-significant interaction between anxiety and defensiveness, $F(1, 76) = 3.46$, $p = .067$, $\eta_p^2 = .044$. A similar 2 × 2 × 2 × (2)

ANOVA of ratings of success yielded only a near-significant main effect of event, $F(1, 76) = 3.42$, $p = .068$, $\eta_p^2 = .043$. Participants in the suppression condition ($M = 5.76$, $SD = 2.10$) reported higher levels of effort than individuals in the nonsuppression condition ($M = 4.55$, $SD = 1.82$). Also, high anxiety individuals (high anxious and defensive high anxious; $M = 5.82$, $SD = 2.13$) reported higher levels of effort than low anxiety individuals; $M = 5.01$, $SD = 2.00$). Notably, repressors reported lower levels of suppression effort ($M = 4.65$, $SD = 2.01$) than all other groups, including low anxious ($M = 5.38$, $SD = 1.95$), high anxious ($M = 5.44$, $SD = 1.83$), and defensive high anxious ($M = 6.58$, $SD = 2.53$) individuals. Although the pattern of button presses suggests that not everyone suppressed (particularly embarrassed) event-related thoughts, all believed that they were relatively successful in not thinking about their proud ($M = 5.82$, $SD = 2.36$) and embarrassed ($M = 6.38$, $SD = 2.61$) events. And although repressors had the lowest levels of both event-related thoughts and suppression effort, they did not rate themselves as more successful at suppressing than other groups.

TABLE 3
Mean change (and standard deviations) in event-related thoughts from the suppression to expression periods ("rebound")

	Instruction	
Anxiety and defensiveness	*Suppression*	*Nonsuppression*
Proud event		
Low anxiety		
Low defensiveness (LA)	−0.81 (2.90)	−0.63 (2.13)
High defensiveness (REP)	−0.38 (2.03)	−1.00 (2.20)
High anxiety		
Low defensiveness (HA)	−0.44 (3.27)	−1.75 (1.67)
High defensiveness (DHA)	0.63 (3.07)	−2.50 (1.00)
Embarrassed event		
Low anxiety		
Low defensiveness (LA)	−1.44 (2.37)	−2.88 (3.31)
High defensiveness (REP)	−0.50 (0.97)	−0.75 (1.04)
High anxiety		
Low defensiveness (HA)	−1.50 (2.28)	−3.63 (6.21)
High defensiveness (DHA)	−1.25 (2.55)	−0.50 (5.07)

Note: LA = low anxious; REP = repressor; HA = high anxious; DHA = defensive high anxious. Positive values represent an increase in event-related thoughts from suppression to expression periods, and negative values represent a decrease.

Rebound of event-related thoughts

Table 3 presents the mean change in event-related thoughts (as indicated by button presses) across the suppression and expression periods for the proud and embarrassed events. Rebound is defined as an increase in event-related thoughts from the suppression to the expression period; in Table 3, positive values represent an increase across the periods and negative values represent a decrease. A 2 (anxiety) × 2 (defensiveness) × (2) (instruction) × (2) (event) mixed-model ANOVA of this data yielded main effects of defensiveness (near significant) and instruction, $F(1, 76) = 3.44$, $p = .068$, $\eta_p^2 = .043$ and $F(1, 76) = 4.67$, $p = .034$, $\eta_p^2 = .058$, respectively. Individuals told to suppress showed less change in event-related thoughts ($M = -.77$, $SD = 1.63$) than individuals not told to suppress ($M = -1.73$, $SD = 2.34$; who reported fewer event-related thoughts during the expression than suppression period). Also high defensive individuals (repressor and defensive high anxious) showed less change in event related thoughts ($M = -0.63$, $SD = 1.58$) than low defensive individuals (low anxious and high anxious; $M = -1.44$, $SD = 2.11$; who also reported fewer thoughts during the expression than suppression period). Overall, there was no rebound effect during the expression period, despite successful suppression (particularly by repressors).

DISCUSSION

Repressors were more successful in suppressing thoughts of an embarrassing autobiographical event than low anxious, high anxious, and defensive high anxious individuals. For the embarrassed event, repressors reported the lowest number of event-related thoughts, rated their suppression attempts as less effortful than all other groups, and showed no rebound. They avoided these thoughts even when not instructed to do so. For the proud event, repressors reported a similar number of thoughts to other groups, and like them, avoided only when instructed. Repressors' different reactions to the proud and embarrassed events confirm that their avoidant processing is engaged by negative self-referent material; in this experiment, an autobiographical memory.

Although we focused on only one negative memory (of an embarrassing event), we believe that repressors' suppression would generalise to other, but perhaps not all, categories of emotionally negative memories. Myers and Brewin (1994) asked repressors to recall childhood memories in response to cues "sorry", "angry", "clumsy", "hurt", and "lonely", and reported that repressors had difficulty recalling memories to all of the cues. In contrast, Davis (1987, experiment 2) asked for memories in response to 10 negative emotion words, and reported that repressors had difficulty recalling memories to only "angry" and "fearful" cues. For different people, the repressive coping style may be engaged by different material/memories. Higgin's (1987; see also Strauman, 1992) self-discrepancy theory predicts, for instance, that memories

(''I was nasty to my mother'') that prime a discrepancy between an individual's self-concept (''I am a nice person'') and their self-evaluative standard or guides (''I should be a nice person'') are associated with emotional discomfort and thus avoided. Individual repressors may be motivated to avoid material that threatens their particular sense of self (Weinberger, 1990).

Repressors' suppression of the embarrassed event is consistent with their response to experimental memory procedures, including autobiographical recall, recall of stories or scenarios, and directed forgetting (Barnier, 2001; Davis, 1987, 1990; Davis & Schwartz, 1987; Krahe, 1999; Myers & Brewin, 1994, 1995; Myers et al., 1998; Newman & Hedberg, 1999). It is consistent also with anxiety biases in memory. Clinically anxious individuals differ substantially from nonanxious controls on procedures that measure attention/encoding or retrieval (e.g., emotional Stroop, dot probe tasks, directed forgetting), especially in response to anxiety-specific stimuli (Cloitre, 1998; MacLeod, 1999).

Repressors as natural suppressors

Repressors' thought suppression suggests that they are highly effective, natural suppressors. They reported few intrusive thoughts of their embarrassed event even when not instructed to suppress. In contrast, low anxious, high anxious, and defensive high anxious participants reported up to 18 intrusive thoughts when not instructed to suppress. Repressors also gave the lowest ratings of suppression effort, which implies that they have a natural suppression style experienced as relatively effortless. Over time and repeated practice, effortful suppression may take the form of a habitual, automatic ''repression'' (Wegner & Zanakos, 1994). Interestingly, repressors did not rate their suppression attempts as more successful than other participants, which suggests that they may lack insight into their avoidance.

It is important to note that, for the embarrassed event, we found main effects of anxiety and defensiveness rather than an interaction between them. Overall, low anxiety individuals (low anxious and repressor) reported fewer event-related thoughts than high anxiety individuals (high anxious and defensive high anxious), and high defensive individuals (repressor and defensive high anxious) reported fewer event-related thoughts than low defensive individuals (low anxious and high anxious). Repressors' performance may be due to anxiety or defensiveness alone, rather than their combination. But numerically, repressors reported the lowest number of event-related thoughts and the distribution data in Table 2 showed a consistent pattern markedly different from other groups. Our failure to detect an interaction is probably due to a lack of power; defensive high anxious individuals are less common in screening samples, but more are needed to clearly separate out the effects of anxiety and defensiveness.

High anxious and defensive high anxious individuals suppressed their embarrassed event when instructed (like repressors). They reported twice as many thoughts of their embarrassing event when not instructed to suppress (unlike repressors). These findings challenge the view that emotional thoughts and memories are invariably difficult to suppress (McNally & Ricciardi, 1996; Wenzlaff & Wegner, 2000). However, the impact of negative emotion may be tempered by the self-relevance of the target thought (Howell & Conway, 1992; Kelly & Kahn, 1994; Renaud & McConnell, 2002). Kelly and Kahn (1994) reported that participants' initial suppression of self-generated intrusive thoughts was followed by diminished expression. They argued that suppressing familiar personal thoughts is less problematic than suppressing other thoughts. Such thoughts or experiences may be easier to suppress, particularly if they have been targeted by avoidance in the past.

Contrary to the predictions of ironic processes theory (Wegner, 1994; Wenzlaff & Wegner, 2000), we did not observe rebound, irrespective of suppression instruction. For low anxious, high anxious, and defensive high anxious individuals, the lack of rebound for their embarrassed event is not surprising; they were less likely to suppress it in the first place. For repressors, the lack of rebound is consistent with our prediction that they may be especially skilled at avoiding a sudden postsuppression increase in thoughts, perhaps by continued vigilance and avoidance (whether automatic or effortful). The lack of rebound could be due to the nature of the targeted material. Rebound is often variable for emotional material, and like suppression success, influenced by self-relevance, familiarity, and even a "rebounding style" (Kelly & Kahn, 1994; Renaud & McConnell, 2002; Rutledge, Hollenberg, & Hancock, 1993).

Repressors' performance may reflect a reporting bias rather than a genuine experience of limited awareness. The thought suppression paradigm relies on a behavioural self-report of subjective experience. Although the number of button presses was significantly correlated with retrospective ratings of thought frequency, it is possible that repressors especially were failing to report what they were actually experiencing. Repressors by definition behave in socially desirable ways (as measured by the MC) and may be highly motivated to meet perceived experimental demands. Research using "bogus pipeline manipulations" suggests instead that they are self-deceivers not other-deceivers (Derakshan & Eysenck, 1999). Rather than simply failing to report intrusions, they may use a different criterion for what counts as an event-related thought. One way to minimise the influence of such factors is to use a procedure that indexes the impact of thought control on incidental recall of avoided material (Anderson & Green, 2001).

Pathways and products of suppression success

Assuming that repressors' reports of event-related thoughts accurately reflect their experience, their seemingly natural suppression style may reflect a relatively inadvertent process similar to that seen in retrieval-induced forgetting

(RIF). In RIF, information or memories that receive retrieval practice (i.e., they are repeatedly retrieved and rehearsed) inhibit the retrieval of items or memories that are related to practised material, but do not receive practice (Anderson, Bjork, & Bjork, 1994). For instance, Barnier, Hung , and Conway (this issue) asked participants to generate up to four autobiographical memories to a number of positive, negative, and neutral category cues. During a retrieval-practice phase, participants practiced retrieving a subset of the memories from each category cue. On a final recall test, participants recalled more practised than unpractised memories from the same category cues. Repressors may focus on (and in effect practice) positive memories at the expense of negative memories, which would decrease the accessibility of negative memories. This is consistent with Davis' (1987, 1990; Davis & Schwartz, 1987; see also Newman & Hedberg, 1999) finding that repressors recalled more positive than negative autobiographical memories from childhood, and Boden and Baumeister's (1997) finding that repressors distracted themselves from an unpleasant film by thinking of pleasant thoughts and memories. Repressors' focus on positive rather than negative memories may begin as an effortful strategy, but become habitual and effortless over time. Indeed, based on Howell and Conway's (1992) finding that individuals are less likely to report negative thought intrusions when they are in a positive mood, repressors may automatically lessen the accessibility of unwanted negative thoughts by simply focusing on positive memories that engender a positive mood.

Both the findings and limitations of this research raise questions for future research on individual differences in thought and memory management. Repressors may be good suppressors because the autobiographical memories they selected and we targeted for suppression were the focus of avoidance in the past; in other words, repressors may have chosen thoughts that they knew they could control. This is one difficulty of using personally generated rather than experimentally controlled material. However, repressors may be much less likely to avoid neutral, low self-relevant targets. It is unclear also whether repressors are avoiding their memory of an event or simply their emotional reaction to it. Schimmack and Hartmann (1997) argued that the repressive coping style influences the experience of emotions rather than the accessibility of memories. Most research has focused on repressors' memory performance rather than considered the extent to which emotional inhibition renders cognitive inhibition more likely (Koutstaal & Schacter, 1997). Notably, our two versions of the suppression instruction, which targeted either emotions or the entire event, had similar effects.

In summary, this experiment highlights important individual differences in the management of (particularly negative) memories. Our results reinforce previous findings that repressors use inhibitory strategies to regulate their awareness of thoughts and memories they find threatening or uncomfortable. Repressors appear to be talented, natural suppressors, at least in the laboratory.

Future research should tell us how repressors use this characteristic style to manage awareness of information in everyday life.

REFERENCES

Abramowitz, J. S., Tolin, D. F., & Street, G. P. (2001). Paradoxical effects of thought suppression: A meta-analysis of controlled studies. *Clinical Psychology Review, 21*, 683–703.

Anderson, M. C., Bjork, R. A., & Bjork, E. L. (1994). Remembering can cause forgetting: Retrieval dynamics in long-term memory. *Journal of Experimental Psychology: Learning, Memory, and Cognition, 20*, 1063–1087.

Anderson, M. C., & Green, C. (2001). Suppressing unwanted memories by executive control. *Nature, 410*, 366–369.

Barnier, A. J. (2001, July). *Individual differences in remembering and forgetting: Repressive copers' avoidance of negative, self-referent information.* Paper presented at the 3rd International Conference on Memory, Valencia, Spain.

Barnier, A. J., Hung, L., & Conway, M. A. (this issue). Retrieval-induced forgetting of emotional and unemotional autobiographical memories. *Cognition and Emotion, 18*, 457–477.

Bjork, R. A. (1989). Retrieval inhibition as an adaptive mechanism in human memory. In H. L. Roediger III & F. I. M. Craik (Eds.), *Varieties of memory and consciousness* (pp. 309–330). Hillsdale, NJ: Erlbaum.

Bjork, E. L., Bjork, R. A., & Anderson, M. C. (1998). Varieties of goal-directed forgetting. In J. M. Golding & C. M. MacLeod (Eds.), *Intentional forgetting: Interdisciplinary approaches* (pp. 139–172). Mahwah, NJ: Lawrence Erlbaum.

Boden, J. M., & Baumeister, R. F. (1997). Repressive coping: Distraction using pleasant thoughts and memories. *Journal of Personality and Social Psychology, 73*, 45–62.

Bonnano, G. A., Davis, P. J., Singer, J. L., & Schwartz, G. E. (1991). The repressor personality and avoidant information processing: A dichotic listening study. *Journal of Research in Personality, 25*, 386–401.

Brewin, C. R. (2001). Memory processes in posttraumatic stress disorder. *International Review of Psychiatry, 13*, 159–163.

Cloitre, M. (1998). Intentional forgetting and clinical disorders. In J. M. Golding & C. M. MacLeod (Eds.), *Intentional forgetting: Interdisciplinary approaches* (pp. 395–412). Mahwah, NJ: Lawrence Erlbaum.

Conway, M. A., & Pleydell-Pearce, C. W. (2000). On the construction of autobiographical memories in a self memory system. *Psychological Review, 107*, 261–288.

Crowne, D. P., & Marlowe, D. A. (1964). *The approval motive: Studies in evaluative dependence.* New York: Wiley.

Dalgleish, T., Mathews, A., & Wood, J. (1999). Inhibition processes in cognition and emotion: A special case? In T. Dalgleish & M. Power (Eds.), *Handbook of cognition and emotion* (pp. 243–265). Chichester, UK: John Wiley.

Davis, P. J. (1987). Repression and the inaccessibility of affective memories. *Journal of Personality and Social Psychology, 53*, 585–593.

Davis, P. J. (1990). Repression and the inaccessibility of emotional memories. In J. L. Singer (Ed.), *Repression and dissociation: Implications for personality theory, psychopathology, and health* (pp. 387–404). Chicago: University of Chicago Press.

Davis, P. J., & Schwartz, G. E. (1987). Repression and the inaccessibility of affective memories. *Journal of Personality and Social Psychology, 52*, 155–162.

Derakshan, N., & Eysenck, M. W. (1997). Repression and repressors: Theoretical and experimental approaches. *European Psychologist, 2*, 235–246.

Derakshan, N., & Eysenck, M. W. (1999). Are repressors self-deceivers or other-deceivers? *Cognition and Emotion*, *13*, 1–17.

Derakshan, N., & Eysenck, M. W. (2001). Effects of focus of attention on physiological, behavioural, and reported state anxiety in repressors, low anxious, high-anxious, and defensive high-anxious individuals. *Anxiety, Stress, and Coping*, *14*, 285–299.

Erdelyi, M. H. (1990). Repression, reconstruction, and defense: History and integration of the psychoanalytic and experimental frameworks. In J. L. Singer (Ed.), *Repression and dissociation: Implications for personality theory, psychopathology, and health* (pp. 1–31). Chicago: University of Chicago Press.

Eysenck, M. W. (2000). A cognitive approach to trait anxiety. *European Journal of Personality*, *14*, 463–476.

Freud, S. (1957). Repression. In J. Strachey (Ed. & Trans.) and C. M. Baines (Trans.), *The standard edition of the complete psychological works of Sigmund Freud* (Vol. 14, pp. 147–165). London: Hogarth Press. (Original work published 1915)

Higgins, E. T. (1987). Self-discrepancy: A theory relating self and affect. *Psychological Review*, *94*, 319–340.

Howell, A., & Conway, M. (1992). Mood and the suppression of positive and negative self-referent thoughts. *Cognitive Therapy and Research*, *16*, 535–555.

Kelly, A., & Kahn, J. H. (1994). Effects of suppression of personal intrusive thoughts. *Journal of Personality and Social Psychology*, *66*, 998–1006.

Kihlstrom, J. F., & Schacter, D. L. (1995). Functional disorders of autobiographical memory. In A. Baddeley, B. A. Wilson, & F. Watts (Eds.), *Handbook of memory disorders* (pp. 337–364). London: Wiley.

Koutstaal, W., & Schacter, D. L. (1997). Intentional forgetting and voluntary thought suppression: Two potential methods for coping with childhood trauma. In L. Dickstein & M. B. Riba (Eds.), *American Psychiatric Press review of psychiatry* (Vol. 16, pp. II79–II121). Washington, DC: American Psychiatric Press.

Krahe, B. (1999). Repression and coping with the threat of rape. *European Journal of Personality*, *13*, 15–26.

MacLeod, C. (1999). Anxiety and anxiety disorders. In T. Dalgleish & M. Power (Eds.), *Handbook of cognition and emotion* (pp. 447–477). New York: John Wiley.

Markowitz, L. J., & Borton, J. L. (2002). Suppression of negative self-referent and neutral thoughts: A preliminary investigation. *Behavioural and Cognitive Psychotherapy*, *30*, 271–277.

McAdams, D. P. (2001). The psychology of life stories. *Review of General Psychology*, *5*, 100–122.

McNally, R.J. (2003). *Remembering trauma*. Cambridge, MA: Harvard University Press.

McNally, R. J., & Ricciardi, J. N. (1996). Suppression of negative and neutral thoughts. *Behavioural and Cognitive Psychotherapy*, *24*, 17–25.

Myers, L. B., & Brewin, C. R. (1994). Recall of early experience and the repressive coping style. *Journal of Abnormal Psychology*, *103*, 288–292.

Myers, L. B., & Brewin, C. R. (1995). Repressive coping and the recall of emotional material. *Cognition and Emotion*, *9*, 637–642.

Myers, L. B., Brewin, C. R., & Power, M. J. (1998). Repressive coping and the directed forgetting of emotional material. *Journal of Abnormal Psychology*, *107*, 141–148.

Newman, L. S., & Hedberg, D. A. (1999). Repressive coping and the inaccessibility of negative autobiographical memories: Converging evidence. *Personality and Individual Differences*, *27*, 45–53.

Newman, L. S., & McKinney, L. C. (2002). Repressive coping and threat avoidance: An idiographic Stroop study. *Personality and Social Psychology Bulletin*, *28*, 409–422.

Rassin, E., Merckelbach, H., & Muris, P. (2000). Paradoxical and less paradoxical effects of thought suppression: A critical review. *Clinical Psychology Review*, *20*, 973–995.

Renaud, J. M., & McConnell, A. R. (2002). Organization of the self-concept and the suppression of self-relevant thoughts. *Journal of Experimental Social Psychology*, *38*, 79–86.

Rutledge, P. C., Hollenberg, D., & Hancock, R. A. (1993). Individual difference in the Wegner rebound effect: Evidence for a moderator variable in thought rebound following thought suppression. *Psychological Reports*, *72*, 867–880.

Schimmack, U., & Hartmann, K. (1997). Individual differences in the memory representation of emotional episodes: Exploring the cognitive processes in repression. *Journal of Personality and Social Psychology*, *75*, 1064–1079.

Singer, J. A., & Salovey, P. (1993). *The remembered self.* New York: The Free Press.

Spielberger, C. D., Gorsuch, R. L., Lushene, R., Vagg, P. R., & Jacobs, G. A. (1983). *Manual for the State-Trait Anxiety Inventory*. Palo Alto, CA: Consulting Psychologists Press.

Strauman, T. J. (1992). Self-guides, autobiographical memory, and anxiety and dysphoria: Toward a cognitive model of vulnerability to emotional distress. *Journal of Abnormal Psychology*, *101*, 87–95.

Tabachnick, B. G., & Fidell, L. S. (1996). *Using multivariate statistics* (3rd ed.). New York: HarperCollins.

Vetere, A., & Myers, L. B. (2002). Repressive coping style and adult romantic attachment style: Is there a relationship? *Personality and Individual Differences*, *32*, 799–807.

Wegner, D. M. (1994). Ironic processes of mental control. *Psychological Review*, *101*, 34–52.

Wegner, D. M., Schneider, D. J., Carter, S. R., & White, T. L. (1987). Paradoxical effects of thought suppression. *Journal of Personality and Social Psychology*, *53*, 5–13.

Wegner, D. M., & Zanakos, S. (1994). Chronic thought suppression. *Journal of Personality*, *62*, 615–640.

Weinberger, D. A. (1990). The construct validity of the repressive coping style. In J. L. Singer (Ed.), *Repression and dissociation: Implications for personality theory, psychopathology, and health* (pp. 337–386). Chicago: University of Chicago Press.

Weinberger, D. A., Schwartz, G. E., & Davidson, R. J. (1979). Low-anxious, high-anxious, and repressive coping styles: Psychometric patterns and behavioral responses to stress. *Journal of Abnormal Psychology*, *88*, 369–380.

Wenzlaff, R. M., & Wegner, D. M. (2000). Thought suppression. *Annual Review of Psychology*, *51*, 59–91.

COGNITION AND EMOTION, 2004, *18* (4), 533–558

Self-induced memory distortions and the allocation of processing resources at encoding and retrieval

Matthew S. Shane and Jordan B. Peterson

University of Toronto, Canada

The present study evaluated the possibility that memory distortions characteristic of repression are due, at least in part, to the reduced allocation of processing resources to unwanted or threatening information. Such reduced processing could occur early, during encoding processes, or conversely, could occur later, during more elaborative, or retrieval-based processes. Repressors and nonrepressors completed a free recall task, which included positively, negatively, and neutrally valenced words, and also completed a go/no-go task previously designed to evaluate the willingness to allocate processing resources to both positive and negative contingent feedback, at encoding, and at retrieval. Results indicated that repressors did evidence reduced memory for negative, but not positive or neutral words, on the free recall task. Repressors also manifested reduced allocation of additional processing resources toward negative contingent feedback as compared to nonrepressors. Finally, the allocation of processing resources at retrieval, but not at encoding, was found to mediate the relationship between participant's self-deceptive enhancement scores and the number of negative words recalled. These results support a model of repression based on motivated attempts to strategically avoid cognitively processing aversive information.

In a recent review of the literature, Mazzoni (2002) suggested that distortions of memory could be conveniently classified into one of two groups. *Naturally occurring distortions* were those that occurred as a result of the inherent frailty of human memory, such as proactive and retroactive interference and primacy and recency effects. *Suggestion-dependent distortions*, in contrast, were those that occurred as a result of external suggestion, such as leading questions or various forms of misinformation. Although the distinction between these two distortion types seems valuable, in both cases the memorial inaccuracies appear,

Correspondence should be addressed to Jordan B. Peterson, Department of Psychology, University of Toronto, 100 St. George St., Toronto, Ontario, Canada, M5S 3G3; e-mail: peterson@psych.utoronto.ca

This research was supported by the Social Sciences and Humanities Research Council of Canada, and by a Connaught Grant from the University of Toronto. We gratefully acknowledge Jonah Hershberg's help in the data collection.

http://www.tandf.co.uk/journals/pp/02699931.html DOI:10.1080/02699930341000437

or are considered, unintentional or involuntary. That is, an underlying assumption of this dual classification system is that distortions of memory occur despite the will of the individual to create an accurate long-term representation of reality.

It is not clear, however, that individuals are universally motivated to represent their environment in an entirely unbiased and veridical fashion. Rather, memorial representations of reality appear frequently influenced by self-serving motives (e.g., Conway & Ross, 1984; Levine, 1997; McFarland & Alvaro, 2000; McFarland & Buehler, 1997, 1998; Ross & Wilson, 2002; Safer & Keuler, 2002; Wilson & Ross, 2001). The existence of such motivated influences suggests that a third type of memory distortion, *self-induced distortions*, also affect how reality is represented in memory systems. Freud (1901/1957) strongly believed that individuals were capable of manipulating their memory processing, and suggested that unwanted thoughts could be actively repressed into the unconscious, where they would lie outside the reach of conscious recollection. Such repressive mechanisms were theorised to serve an ego-protection function, reducing the level of stress and anxiety that conscious recollection of the threatening or unwanted thoughts would otherwise cause. Consistent with this notion, reports of significant gaps in memories for major traumatic life experiences, including childhood abuse, have been documented in numerous studies (e.g., Feldman-Summers & Pope, 1994; Loftus, Polonsky, & Fullilove, 1994; Tromp, Koss, Figueredo, & Tharan, 1995; Williams, 1994). Furthermore, recent theorists have noted that posttraumatic stress disorder (PTSD) is generally characterised by reduced memory for the contextual and emotional details surrounding the events that led to the onset of the disorder (e.g., Brewin, 2001; Foa, Molnar, & Cashman, 1995; Harvey & Bryant, 1999).

Although the memory distortions noted in victims of childhood abuse or PTSD patients may be particularly severe, such distortions do not appear limited to clinical populations. Rather, self-induced memory distortions appear to occur regularly in the general population, in the service of a variety of self-serving motives, including "mood repair" (McFarland & Buehler, 1998), justification of current goals and needs (Conway & Ross, 1984; Levine, 1997; McFarland & Alvaro, 2000; Safer & Keuler, 2002), regulation of affective experiences (McFarland & Buehler, 1997), and maintenance of current self-concepts (Ross & Wilson, 2002; Wilson & Ross, 2001). McFarland and Buehler (1997, 1998) have demonstrated, for instance, that individuals currently experiencing a negative mood may manifest a "mood-incongruent bias", whereby they recall more positive information than negative information. These authors have suggested that such a mood-incongruent bias may be motivated through an active attempt to "repair" the current negative mood state. Consistent with this notion, there does not appear to be a similar mood-incongruent bias when individuals are experiencing a positive mood state.

Evidence of self-induced memory distortions are not limited to memory search, but also appear to affect the reconstruction of existing memory traces (Bahrick, Hall, & Berger, 1996; McDonald & Hirt, 1997; McFarland & Alvaro, 2000; Safer & Keuler, 2002). Bahrick et al. (1996), for example, demonstrated that students strategically overestimated their previous performance in school, and proposed an affect-regulation hypothesis, whereby the memory enhancements served to promote higher levels of positive affect. Consistent with this notion, the level of overestimation was inversely proportionate to the level of original performance. Thus, individuals at more apparent risk for negative mood states demonstrated larger memory distortions. In contrast, Safer and Keuler (2002) have provided evidence for a different type of overestimation distortion, whereby individuals overestimated previous levels of distress after participating in therapeutic sessions. Similar overestimations of previous distress levels have been noted with regard to study skills acquisition (Conway & Ross, 1984), and growth after trauma (McFarland & Alvaro, 2000), and have been theorised to justify participation in the treatment, enhance current mood and provide evidence of improvement over time (Conway & Ross, 1984).

Individual differences in self-induced memory distortions

Operating under the assumption that some individuals are more motivated to distort their memories, researchers have found it fruitful to investigate the use of repressive mechanisms from an individual differences perspective. As already noted, PTSD patients and victims of childhood abuse appear particularly likely to utilise these mechanisms. Additionally, however, personality researchers have begun investigating repression, per se, as a trait construct. To this end, Weinberger, Schwartz, and Davidson (1979) defined repressors as individuals who scored below the mean on the Taylor Manifest Anxiety Scale (TMAS: Taylor, 1953), and above the mean on the Marlow-Crowne Social Desirability Scale (MCSD: Crowne & Marlow, 1960). Generally, a preoccupation with the view of others is indicative of elevated levels of anxiety. Thus, the combination of high MCSD scores and low TMAS scores suggests dissociation between actual and subjective levels of experienced anxiety. In keeping with this suggestion, there is good empirical evidence demonstrating that repressors consistently manifest higher physiological reactivity and slower physiological recovery to aversive or threatening stimuli, in comparison to high and low anxious individuals (e.g., heart rate: Fuller, 1992; cortisol: Brown et al., 1996; endorphins: Jamner, Schwartz, & Leigh, 1988). Moreover, repressors appear to be at higher risk for somatic diseases, including cardiovascular disease and cancer (Lane & Schwartz, 1987).

In contrast to evidence demonstrating repressors' increased sensitivity to negative or threatening information, evidence of self-induced memory distortion in repressors has been less consistent. Myers and Brewin (1995) required repressors, high anxious and low anxious individuals to learn a story containing equal portions of positive and negative information. Repressors recollected significantly fewer negative phrases than both high and low anxious individuals, providing evidence for increased levels of self-induced distortions, but were not characterised by differential recall of positive or neutral material. Davis (1987) and Davis and Schwartz (1987) demonstrated that self-deceivers were characterised by reduced ability to recall negative autobiographical memories during both free and cued recall tasks (see also Newman & Hedberg, 1999). Similarly, Holtgraves and Hall (1995) showed that repressors demonstrated a reduced ability to remember previous events that were associated with particular negative emotions. Finally, Bonanno, Davis, Singer and Schwartz (1991) used a dichotic listening task to show that repressors manifested poorer memory than non-repressors for threatening words in the to-be-ignored channel. In contrast, both Oldenburg and Kivistoe (2002) and Brosschot, De Ruiter, and Kindt (1999) found no differences between repressors and high/low anxious individuals with regard to memory for threatening, positive or neutral words. One difference between these latter two studies involved the level of self-relevance of the material to be remembered. Thus, one possibility is that repressors only find it necessary to distort their memories regarding highly self-relevant negative information.

The present study sought, in part, to attempt to provide evidence that repressors would exhibit decreased memory, even to negative or threatening information that was not highly self-relevant. To this end, repressors and non-repressors were required to perform a free recall memory task, including an equal number of positive, negative, and neutral words. Reduced memory for negative, but not positive or neutral, words among repressors would support the notion that they attempt to reduce the impact of all negatively valenced information, regardless of its direct self-relevance.

How and when are self-induced distortions created?

Despite considerable research into the existence of memory distortions in repressors, very few studies have attempted to examine the mechanisms underlying repressive processing. Freud's theoretical stance regarding repression highlighted the importance of two processes, one more "conscious", the other more "unconscious" (Freud, 1901/1957). The conscious, more active, process involved refusing to admit to the existence of threatening ideas, impulses or memories that try to emerge from the unconscious, their original source. The unconscious, more passive process involved the tendency of the unconscious to gather about itself ideas, impulses and memories associated with the originally repressed material. Although details regarding how these processes operate were not well elucidated by Freud (a state of affairs which has not improved much to the present day), modern researchers have proposed a number of different mechanisms which may influence memory processing, and which appear broadly akin to Freud's repression hypotheses.

First, in keeping with the notion of unconscious operations, researchers have implicated reduced accessibility to negative information in repressors, which may limit the likelihood that such information will be automatically activated through associative networks (Baddeley, 1999; Baddeley & Hitch, 1994). In support of this notion, Davis (1987) has demonstrated that repressors are slower to report negative autobiographic memories than nonrepressors, and Myers, Brewin, and Power (1998) have reported that repressors are older at the age of their earliest recalled negative memory than nonrepressors. Exactly how this reduced accessibility occurs, however, has not been well established to date. Consistent with evidence from Hansen and Hansen (1988; see also Hansen, Hansen, & Schantz, 1992) suggesting that repressors show reduced intensity of secondary emotions associated with a particular emotional event, Davis (1987) suggested that repressors may have less complex and more isolated memory representations than do nonrepressors. This notion may be true, but in turn simply begs the further question of how this reduced complexity occurs.

Second, in keeping with the notion of a more motivated, controllable repressive process, a number of researchers have theorized that repressors show globally enhanced levels of inhibitory control, and thus are better enabled to inhibit processing of unwanted information (e.g., Bjork, 1989; Bonanno et al., 1991; Hasher & Zacks, 1988; Myers et al., 1998). Evidence in support of this notion comes from studies requiring participants to attend to some stimuli, and ignore other stimuli. Myers et al. (1998), for instance, required repressors and nonrepressors to learn a list of positive and negative words, and after such learning, to forget that list of words and learn another similar list of positive and negative words. In a surprise free recall task in which participants were asked to recall as many words as possible from either list, repressors showed reduced ability to recall negative, but not positive, words from the to-be-forgotten list. Bonanno et al. (1991) reported similar results in a dichotomous listening task, whereby repressors showed reduced interference from, and reduced memory for, threatening words in the to-be-ignored channel than either high or low anxious individuals.

Although these studies are important, there are complications involved with interpreting repression as involving either global enhancement of inhibitory control or global interference with retrieval. First, such interpretations fail to address the time course over which putatively repressive mechanisms might operate. Inhibition of unwanted thoughts could occur early, during attentive or pre attentive processing, and could thus reduce the extent to which unwanted information is processed during encoding (see Bonanno et al., 1991; Dawkins & Furnham, 1989; Hansen & Hansen, 1988; Hock, Krone, & Kaiser, 1996;

Newman & Hedberg, 1999; Schimmack & Hartmann, 1997). Alternatively, inhibition could occur later on, during more elaborative or retrieval-based processes, more directly reducing the likelihood that unwanted information will be retrieved from memory (see Holtgraves & Hall, 1995; Lorig, Singer, Bonanno, Davis, & Schwartz, 1994; Myers et al., 1998). Evidence exists in support of both possibilities. Bonanno et al.'s (1991) work with the dichotic listening task, along with other research demonstrating reduced Stroop interference in repressors (Dawkins & Furnham, 1989), suggests the existence of encoding-based differences between repressors and nonrepressors (see also Newman & Hedberg, 1999). Myers et al. (1998), conversely, suggests the existence of retrieval-based differences, since instructions to inhibit the to-be-forgotten words were not given until after all words were equally encoded (see also Holtgraves & Hall, 1995 and Lorig et al., 1994). Note, however, that repressors only demonstrated reduced memory for threatening to-be-forgotten words, and thus, such reduced memories could have occurred during the encoding stage. It seems plausible to hypothesise that repression might involve both encoding-based, and retrieval-based inhibition, and this suggestion has been made previously (e.g., Holtgraves & Hall, 1995). However, further investigation is required to determine when each type of repressive process will most likely be utilised.

Second, the fact that the repressors in Myers et al. (1998) and Bonanno et al. (1991) showed reduced recall only for threatening to-be-forgotten/ignored words, rather than for all to-be-forgotten/ignored words, also argues against the notion that repressors are characterised by global enhancements in inhibitory control. Rather, it seems that these individuals may be particularly proficient at inhibiting negative or threatening information. Consistent with this notion, Boden and Baumiester (1997) recently demonstrated that repressors may show *increased* accessibility to positive memories, and Fox (1993) has demonstrated that repressors shift attention away from negative stimuli. Repressors may not, then, benefit from enhanced inhibitory control mechanisms, but may simply be more motivated to ignore negative or threatening information, and thus may engage in more strenuous attempts to inhibit such information. Recent research supports such ideas: Holtgraves and Hall (1995) found that repressors showed reduced effort when attempting to retrieve negative memories, and Lorig et al. (1994) demonstrated that repressors showed increased alpha waves (indicative of brain inactivity) when asked to recall distant memories.

The present study attempted to address these issues by requiring participants who performed the free recall task described above to also participate in a procedure that the present authors have previously shown to evaluate the distribution of attentional resources toward positive and negative information, both at the time of encoding and at the time of retrieval (Shane & Peterson, 2004, in press; see also Newman, Patterson, Howland, & Nichols, 1990). The procedure is a trial and error learning task, during which the participant must attempt to learn when to press, and when not to press, a spacebar on a computer. Different two-digit numbers are used as stimulus cues, and contingent positive and negative feedback is supplied after every button-press response. The length of time that this feedback remains onscreen is self-regulated, in that the participant must repress the spacebar after feedback is supplied in order to progress to the next trial.

The measure of attentional distribution garnered from this task, termed "reflective preference" (RP), is defined as *time spent attending to negative feedback / time spent attending to positive feedback*, and was designed to provide an estimate of the tendency or willingness to explore information signalling failure in goal-directed behaviour. Since RP is a ratio measure, it provides control for overall reflection time, and thus indicates the extent to which individuals allocate additional processing resources when feedback signalling error in goal-directed behaviour occurs. The trial and error learning task described above allows for two separate measures of RP: postresponse reflective preference (PostRP), and preresponse reflective preference (PreRP).

PostRP is calculated as the ratio of time spent reflecting on contingent negative feedback to time spent reflecting on contingent positive feedback. Thus, high levels of PostRP indicate relatively greater attention to negatively valenced feedback. Shafrir and Pascal-Leone (1990) first made use of a similar measure in 8-to-10 year old boys, and demonstrated positive correlations with IQ, and a variety of inductive and deductive tasks. Shane and Peterson (2004) have recently replicated this finding in adults, demonstrating that high levels of PostRP predict superior learning of the stimulus-response contingencies on the trial and error learning task. Most recently, Shane and Peterson (in press) demonstrated lower levels of PostRP (and reduced stimulus-response learning) in repressors, suggesting that these individuals may be characterised by decreased willingness to allocate processing resources toward performance-contingent negative feedback.

PreRP, in contrast, is calculated as the ratio of time paused *before a subsequent* error to time paused *before a subsequent* success. In order to remember a previous experience, the experience must not only be appropriately encoded, but must also be summoned from memory at the appropriate time. Such memories may be explicitly recalled as a consequence of the activation of appropriate associations (Bower, 1981), or conversely, may occur more implicitly, through emotional or physiological reactions to specific stimulus presentations (Damasio, 1994). PreRP was created to index attention allocated to the recollection of such implicit or explicit memories. Any change from zero in average PreRP necessarily indicates a distinction between the nature of correct and incorrect stimuli was made. Higher levels of PreRP (indicating longer pauses before making an error, relative to a correct response), may, therefore, be interpreted as indicating the allocation of additional processing resources toward recollection of a stimulus previously linked with negative feedback. In the same way, lower levels of PreRP (indicating shorter pauses before making an error, relative to a correct response) may be interpreted as indicating an unwillingness to think about and learn from previous negative feedback. Shane and Peterson (2004) have recently demonstrated that PreRP predicts an independent portion of the variance in S-R learning on the trial and error learning test, once PostRP is controlled for.

The present study, then, was predicated on several hypotheses. First, it was hypothesised that repressors would manifest reduced recall of negative, but not positive or neutral words, on the free recall memory task when compared to high and low anxious participants. Second, it was hypothesised that repressors would manifest reduced levels of RP, indicating their reduced willingness to allocate processing resources toward negative information. Previous research has already demonstrated reduced PostRP in repressors (Shane & Peterson, in press), however, PreRP has never been investigated in this population. Reduced levels of PreRP in repressors would indicate reduced willingness to allocate processing resources toward the retrieval of negative information. Third, it was hypothesised that levels of both PostRP and PreRP would predict distortions in participant's recall of the word lists: Individuals who allocate less attention toward negative information at either encoding or retrieval should be characterised by increased memory distortions, demonstrated by reduced memory, particularly for the negative words. Last, it was hypothesised that level of either PostRP or PreRP, or both, would mediate the relationship between repressive tendencies and reduced memory for negative words. That is, decreased allocation of processing resources, at encoding, at retrieval, or at both instances, would be seen as at least partially responsible for the reduced ability of repressors to recall the negative words.

METHOD

Participants

A total of 72 undergraduate psychology students at the University of Toronto participated in the study, in partial fulfilment of a course requirement: 52 participants were female; 20 were male. Their ages ranged from 17 to 28 (mean = 20.35).

Measures

Balanced Inventory of Desirable Responding. The BIDR (Paulhus, 1991) is a 40-item inventory consisting of two 20-item subscales: Self-Deceptive Enhancement (SDE) and Impression Management (IM). SDE assesses defensiveness towards personal weakness (e.g., "I have never doubted my ability as a lover") and a general egoistic or overconfident response bias (e.g., "I am fully in control of my own fate") (Paulhus & John, 1998). IM measures the tendency to make oneself look better by denying socially undesirable behaviour (e.g., ''I never take things that don't belong to me'').[1]

Taylor Manifest Anxiety Scale. The TMAS (Taylor, 1953) is a 20-item true/false, forced-choice questionnaire which has been well validated as a measure of anxiety, and has commonly been utilised in the repressive literature for classification of repressors.

Data analytic strategies. Following Weinberger, Schwartz, and Davidson (1979), most recent research on repression has classified participants as repressive copers in a categorical fashion, based on their pattern of scores on the TMAS and the MCSD. Both of these scales evaluate continuous personality traits, however, and thus, by rights, should be analysed in a continuous manner (Wright, 2003). With these two considerations in mind, we decided to conduct our analyses utilising both categorical and continuous strategies. In the categorical analyses, repressors were compared to nonrepressors in a manner similar to that suggested by Weinberger (1995; see below for description). This analysis allows the present findings to be more directly compared to the previous literature. The continuous analyses should, however, provide a more in-depth investigation into the individual contributions of anxiety and defensiveness on attentional and memory processing.

Categorical classifications. The categorical selection criteria utilised, similar to those suggested by Weinberger (1995), were based on patterns of scores on both the TMAS and the SDE.[1] Participants were classified as repressors if they scored above the median on the SDE and below the median on the TMAS. Repressors were therefore those participants who rated themselves as high on self-deceptive enhancement and low in anxiety—a pattern of self-description suggesting suppression of negative affect. In contrast, nonrepressors were those who scored below the median on SDE, regardless of their TMAS score.[2]

---

[1] Weinberger originally utilised the Marlowe-Crown Social Desirability Index (MCSD) rather than the SDE for participant classification. Furnham, Petrides, and Spencer-Bowdage (2002) have demonstrated that use of either the MCSD or the SDE are valid, and similar, identifiers of individuals who utilise repressive coping styles. We believe, however, that the SDE is a more appropriate measure, due to its ability to separate socially desirable responding from more internally self-enhancing tendencies (Paulhus, 1984, 1986).

[2] Participants scoring above the median on both the SDE and TMAS (n = 12) were not included in the categorical analyses. This group, generally making up a fairly small proportion of the total population, has sometimes been referred to as a ''defensive high anxious group''. Researchers have had difficulty classifying this group as it is somewhat unclear as to whether these individuals are more characteristic of repressors or high anxious individuals. It should be noted that all participants, including those in this ''defensive high anxious'' group, were included in the continuous analyses.

Memory task

Participants were seated in front of a Pentium II computer in a quiet room in the laboratory, and were provided with the following instructions:

> This will be a standard memory test. It will test how well you can remember items in short-term memory, and how well you can transfer them to long-term memory. A list of words is going to be displayed on the computer screen, one at a time. Each word will remain on the screen for 2 seconds, and then will be replaced by the next word. There will be 75 words in all. Your task is to remember as many of the words as you can. Don't worry. Nobody can remember all of the words. However, you will be tested on these words later, so try to remember as many as you can.

Word presentation began when the participant pressed the spacebar. The 75 words were then displayed, in random order, for 2000 ms each. Twenty-five words were positively valenced (e.g., love, brilliant, winner), 25 were negatively valenced (e.g., bleeding, death, ugly), and 25 were neutral (e.g., desk, computer, hair). At no time were participants made aware that the words differed with regard to their valence. With the random presentation order, each word type could appear at any point in the presentation stream. Each word list was matched for word length and frequency based on Kučera and Francis's (1967) standardised tables. The interword interval was 1000 ms. Participants were not allowed to write the words down.

A filler task, composed of five mathematical sequencing tasks, was performed between the presentation of the words and the recall task (to reduce the possibility that the results could be due to primacy or recency effects). The sequencing tasks required participants to find the next three numbers in a presented sequence of numbers, and were made challenging enough so as to require significant mental resources, but simple enough so as to generally allow for an eventual solution. The five sequencing tasks took approximately 5 minutes for participants to complete. If, after 5 minutes, participants were still working on the sequences, they were stopped and instructed to continue on to the next task (the recall task). If they finished before 5 minutes expired, they were asked to wait before continuing on. This was done to ensure that differences in word retention were not due to differences in duration between presentation and recall.

The recall task was performed on the same computer that the words were originally presented on, and participants were asked to type in as many of the words as they could from the presented list. Participants were instructed that they would not be docked for providing incorrect words, but that we were not only interested in the quantity of words generated, but also the accuracy of those generated words. In total, the task required 10 to 12 minutes to complete.

Evaluation of reflective preference

Participant's reflective preference was evaluated through use of a modified version of the trial and error go/no-go learning task used by Shane and Peterson (2004, in press; see also Newman et al., 1990). Ten two-digit numbers (e.g., 15, 24, 38, 47) were presented on-screen, one at a time, and participants were instructed to learn through trial and error which numbers indicated that they should respond (by pressing the spacebar) and which numbers indicated that they should not respond (thus, withholding the keypress). Five numbers were "go" cues, while the other five were "no-go" cues. Following correct responses, the stimulus number was immediately replaced by the message "Correct. Good job!", a high-pitched tone (625 Hz) was played through the computer speaker, and one token was awarded. Following incorrect responses, the message "Wrong. Too bad!" appeared, a low-pitched tone (125 Hz) was played, and one token was deducted. The length of time that this feedback remained on-screen was self-regulated—that is, the participant had to repress the spacebar to continue onto the next trial. Participants were not informed that their response times were being recorded. No feedback was provided—and, therefore, no second response was required—when the participant did not respond to the stimulus. Each number was presented nine times in pseudo-random order, for a total of 90 experimental trials. In the case of a nonresponse, the stimulus remained on the screen for 3000 ms; the intertrial interval was 1000 ms.

After being provided with task instructions, participants completed 10 practice trials, using 01 and 02 as stimuli. If a participant did not appear to understand the task during the practice trials, additional instruction was provided to ensure all participants began the real trials with the same level of understanding.

Procedure

All participants completed the study in the same order, in order to reduce the likelihood of interference effects on the memory test. Participants completed the personality measures first, followed by the presentation of the word list, the mathematical filler task, the recall task, and finally, the attentional allocation task. Upon completion of the study, participants were fully debriefed, provided with their experimental credit, and allowed to leave.

RESULTS

Participant characteristics

Means and standard deviations of participants' personality, and reflection data are displayed in Table 1. Participants' TMAS scores and SDE scores were correlated, $r = -.22$, $p = .04$, consistent with previous research utilising self-enhancement and anxiety measures. The number of total words recalled ranged from 4 to 40, with a mean of 16.53, or approximately 22% of the original word

TABLE 1
Mean (and standard deviations) for SDE, TMAS, PostRP, and PreRP for repressors and nonrepressors

Group	*SDE*	*TMAS*	*PostRP*[a]	*PreRP*	*Total words recalled*
All participants ($N = 72$)	4.21 (0.79)	9.13 (3.19)	1.14 (0.60)	1.31 (0.27)	16.79 (7.09)
Nonrepressors ($n = 36$)	3.60 (0.41)	10.00 (2.94)	1.15 (0.60	1.37 (0.28)	18.60 (7.70)
Repressors ($n = 24$)	4.75 (0.52)	6.42 (1.56)	1.23 (0.66)	1.23 (0.28)	15.25 (6.46)

SDE = Self-Deceptive Enhancement; TMAS = Anxiety; PostRP = Post-response reflective preference; PreRP = Preresponse reflective preference.
[a] Only 23 repressors were included in the PostRP data.

list. Independent *t*-tests determined that repressors had significantly higher SDE scores, $t(58) = 9.52, p < .001$, and lower TMAS scores, $t(58) = -5.47, p < .001$, than nonrepressors.

Recall of positive, negative, and neutral words

Categorical analyses: Repressors vs. nonrepressors. Memory data was not collected for one nonrepressor, due to their having to leave before the memory test could be performed. Figure 1 displays the mean number of positive, negative, and neutral words recalled by each group. A 2 (group) × 3 (word type) mixed ANOVA design with word type as a within-subject variable and group as a between subject variable yielded a significant main effect of word type, $F(2, 57) = 5.61$, $p = .005$. Planned comparisons indicated that negative words were recalled more often than either positive words, $t(58) = 4.22$, $p < .001$, or neutral words $t(58) = 1.88, p > .06$. Neutral words were not recalled to a greater extent than positive words, $t(58) = 1.68$, $p = .10$. The main effect of group trended toward significance, $F(1, 57) = 3.14$, $p = .08$, but must be interpreted alongside the word type × group interaction, which also emerged as significant, $F(2, 57) = 3.56, p = .03$.

To dissect the interaction term, planned comparisons were conducted for recall of negative, positive and neutral words, respectively. Only the planned comparison for recall of negative words reached significance [negative: $t(57) = 2.79$, $p = .007$; neutral: $t(57) = 0.58$, positive: $t(57) = 0.74$, *ps* > .4] indicating that repressors recalled less negative, but not less positive or neutral, words than nonrepressors. It should be noted, however, that the repressors were characterised by a reasonably consistent, although nonsignificant, pattern of reduced recall for all three word types.

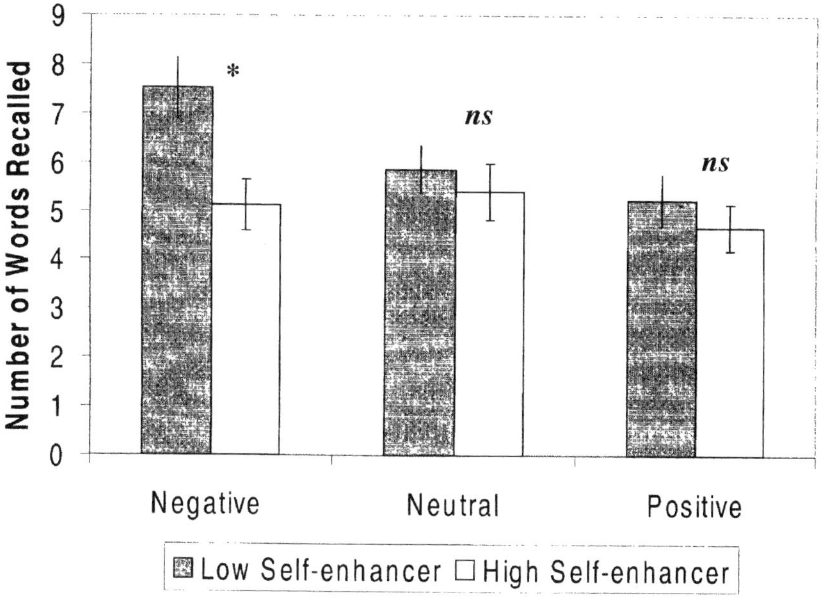

Figure 1. Number of negative, positive, and neutral words recalled by repressors and nonrepressors on a free recall task. $*p < .01$.

A number of additional exploratory analyses were undertaken, to see if the pattern of memory distortion in repressors could be better differentiated. First, we computed a *recall of negative words-recall of positive words* difference score to investigate the possibility that repressors would show a memory bias toward positive information. This analysis yielded a highly significant result, $t(57) = 2.52$, $p = .02$, indicating most directly that repressors (mean difference score = 0.50, $SD = 2.38$) manifested considerable favouritism for positively valenced words over that of nonrepressors (mean difference score = 2.29, $SD = 2.87$). Similarly, we computed a *recall of positive/negative words-recall of neutral words* difference score, to investigate the possibility that repressors may also demonstrate a preference for neutral words, over either type of emotionally valent word. A Levene's test demonstrated unequal variance distributions between the two groups, however, the analysis still emerged as significant with this taken into account, $t(57) = 2.06$, $p = .04$. Thus, repressors may also be characterised by decreased memory for emotional content (repressors: Mean difference score = 4.42, $SD = 3.49$; nonrepressors: Mean difference score = 6.89, $SD = 5.71$).

Last, we investigated the possibility that repressors may evidence a reduced number of false recalls of negative words than nonrepressors. Such reduced false recall may be predicted if repressors make fewer associations to the negative stimuli. A 2 (group) × 3 (false word type) repeated-measures ANOVA did not reveal the predicted interaction, $F(2, 56) = 0.90$, $p > .4$. A main effect of group trended toward significance, $F(1, 57) = 3.36$, $p = .07$, however, suggesting that repressors ($M = 1.75$, $SD = 1.82$) may have made somewhat fewer false recall errors than repressors ($M = 2.80$; $SD = 2.36$), regardless of word valence.

Continuous analyses: SDE and TMAS. In order to more accurately characterise the continuous nature of the SDE and TMAS scales, and to better investigate the individual contributions of each personality trait to the formation of self-induced distortions, we also conducted hierarchical regression analyses using SDE and TMAS (and their interaction) as predictors of memory for positive, negative, and neutral words. A significant SDE × TMAS interaction would be most akin to the demonstration of differences between repressors and nonrepressors in the categorical analyses. Four separate regression models were considered: one for each word type. Initial collinearity between the measures and the interaction term were reduced by centering the predictors before entering them in the regression model. SDE and TMAS were entered in block 1, and the SDE × TMAS interaction term was entered in block 2. Table 2 displays the results of the four regression analyses. As can be seen, the predicted SDE ×

TABLE 2
Results of the regression analyses

Variable	*Standardised coefficient (β)*	*T-value*	*p-value*
Negative recall			
SDE	−.335	−2.90	.005
TMAS	.034	0.29	.772
Total model: $r = .34$, $p = .01$			
Positive recall			
SDE	−.025	−0.20	.840
TMAS	−.017	−0.14	.890
Total model: $r = .03$, $p > .90$			
Neutral recall			
SDE	−.091	−0.74	.460
TMAS	−.130	−1.06	.291
Total model: $r = .14$, $p > .40$			
Total recall			
SDE	−.198	−1.64	.107
TMAS	−.044	−0.37	.714
Total model: $r = .20$, $p > .20$			

Note: The SDE × TMAS interaction was not included in any model in which it did not reach significance ($ps < .05$).

TMAS interaction did not reach significance in any of the models, nor did TMAS alone, suggesting that anxiety level may not be as strong a predictor of memorial distortions as defensiveness. Rather, SDE was the sole predictor of participant's recall, reaching a significant level of prediction for recall of negative, but not positive or neutral words. Specifically, higher levels of SDE tended to predict lower recall of negative words. Again, it should be noted that there was a trend toward SDE predicting overall memory recall, however, this prediction did not quite reach significance.

As with the categorical analyses, we also conducted regression analyses to predict the *recall of negative words-recall of positive words* difference score, and the *recall of negative and positive words-recall of neutral words* difference score, to attempt to better characterise the relationship between the personality traits and memory biases. Consistent with the previously reported findings, SDE, $\beta = -.353$, $p = .003$, but not TMAS, $\beta = .054$, or the SDE $\times$ TMAS interaction term, $\beta = -.033$, was significantly predictive of the number of negative minus positive words recalled (indicative of a positivity bias). No significant results emerged regarding the negative/positive-neutral difference score.

Allocation of attentional resources at encoding and retrieval

PostRP was calculated by determining the ratio of time that negative feedback versus positive feedback was left on-screen during the trial and error learning task, and thus indexed the increased processing resources allocated to negative information during initial encoding of that information. PreRP, in contrast, was calculated by determining the ratio of time paused before making a mistake to time paused before making a correct response, and thus indexed the increased processing resources allocated to negative information during the retrieval of that information from memory. One repressor's PostRP score was over 3 standard deviations above the mean, and over 1 standard deviation above that of the next closest participant. Based on this fact, and exploratory observations of the dataset, it was deemed more accurate to remove this participant's score for all analyses dealing with PostRP.

Consistent with the previous literature (Shane & Peterson, 2004, in press), initial analyses determined that PostRP and PreRP were uncorrelated ($r = .05$, $p > .70$). Also consistent with this literature, PostRP was highly predictive of rate of learning on the trial and error learning task ($r = .62$, $p < .001$), while PreRP was also predictive of such learning for those individuals who were low in PostRP ($r = .49$, $p = .002$). These results have been reported elsewhere (Shane & Peterson, 2004) and thus interested readers are directed therein. For the present article, however, we were particularly interested in the relationship between repression, RP and memory for the positive, negative and neutral words. First, we report the relationship between repression and RP; next we will report the RP-memory distortion relationship.

Repression and RP. To test the specific hypotheses of the study, separate planned comparisons were conducted to determine whether repressors manifested lower PostRP and/or PreRP than nonrepressors. Columns 4 and 5 of Table 1 display the means and standard deviations of PostRP and PreRP, respectively. Consistent with predictions, repressors did exhibit reduced levels of PreRP, $t(58) = 1.85$, $p = .03$, indicating a reduced allocation of processing resources toward the retrieval of negative information. No significant differences were found for PostRP ($p > .60$), suggesting that repressors in the present sample were not characterised by reduced allocation of processing toward the encoding of this information.

Regression was also conducted utilising SDE and TMAS as continuous variables, to attempt to better understand the individual relationships of each personality trait to the RP measures. Separate models were investigated for PreRP and PostRP. The centred SDE and TMAS scores were entered in block 1, and the SDE × TMAS interaction term was entered in block 2. Mirroring the results from the memory data, SDE, $\beta = -.395$, $p < .001$, was the only significant predictor of PreRP (TMAS, $\beta = .077$; SDE × TMAS, $\beta = .052$). Thus, once again it appeared that defensiveness, rather than anxiety level, may be more indicative of behavioural manifestations of repression. The PostRP regression model did not reach significance.

RP and memory distortion. Columns 2–6 of Table 3 display the zero order correlations between PostRP, PreRP, and the various measures of memory evaluated in the present study. As can be seen, both RP measures correlated significantly with overall recall, and recall for both negative and positive, but not neutral words. Additionally, both PostRP and PreRP correlated significantly with the difference between emotional and nonemotional words recalled. That

TABLE 3

Correlational matrix comparing relationship between both RP measures, and memory for the positive, negative, and neutral words on the free recall task

Group	*Positive*	*Negative*	*Neutral*	*Total*	*Pos-Neg*	*Pos/Neg-Neut*
PostRP ($n = 58$)	.28**	.28**	.24**	.34**	.07	.23*
PreRP ($n = 59$)	.26**	.38***	.16	.34***	.18	.32**

*$p > .07$; **$p > .05$; ***$p > .01$.

is, individuals who manifested higher levels of either PostRP or PreRP demonstrated an increased ability to recall either positive or negative words, in comparison to neutral words. Thus, increased processing of negative information at either encoding or retrieval appears to increase recall ability, particularly for emotionally valent information.

To better understand the individual contribution of PostRP and PreRP to recall ability, hierarchical regression analyses were also performed to predict recall of positive, negative, neutral, and total words. A PostRP × PreRP interaction term was calculated by centering the two RP measures (to reduce potential collinearity), and multiplying the two centred variables together. PostRP and PreRP were entered in the first block, and the PostRP × PreRP interaction term in the second block. Table 4 displays the results of these regression analyses. As can be seen, PostRP and PreRP both contributed individually to the recall of negative words and to the total number of words recalled. PostRP also predicted recall of positive words, whereas neither PostRP nor PreRP predicted recall of neural words. The interaction term did not reach significance in any of the regression analyses, although it came closest for the recall of negative words ($\beta = .191$, $p = .14$).

TABLE 4
Results of the regression analyses

Variable	*Standardised coefficient (β)*	*T-value*	*p-value*
Negative recall			
PostRP	.229	2.05	.047
PreRP	.329	2.95	.004
Total model: $r = .43$, $p < .001$			
Positive recall			
PostRP	.244	2.11	.039
PreRP	.214	1.84	.070
Total model: $r = .35$, $p = .01$			
Neutral recall			
PostRP	.217	1.82	.074
PreRP	.115	0.965	.338
Total model: $r = .26$, $p = .09$			
Total recall			
PostRP	.295	2.61	.123
PreRP	.001	0.008	.994
Total model: $r = .34$, $p < .001$			

Note: The PostRP × PreRP interaction was not included in any model because it did not ever reach significance ($ps > .1$).

An introductory model of repression

Self-deceptive enhancement → PreRP → Memory distortion. Additional hierarchical analyses were conducted in order to investigate the possibility that PreRP mediated the relationship between repressive tendencies and memory distortions. Such mediation would provide evidence to support the notion that PreRP is causally related to repressor's enhanced levels of memory distortion. Specifically, we were interested in testing a model of repression whereby self-deceptive enhancement caused distortions in memory to occur, through the reduced use of RP. Although we originally believed that both PreRP and PostRP might act as causal mechanisms, we did not investigate the potential mediating effects of PostRP in the present sample because repressors failed to evidence heightened levels. SDE scores were entered in the first block, followed by PreRP in the second block, in order to predict both recall of negative words, and recall

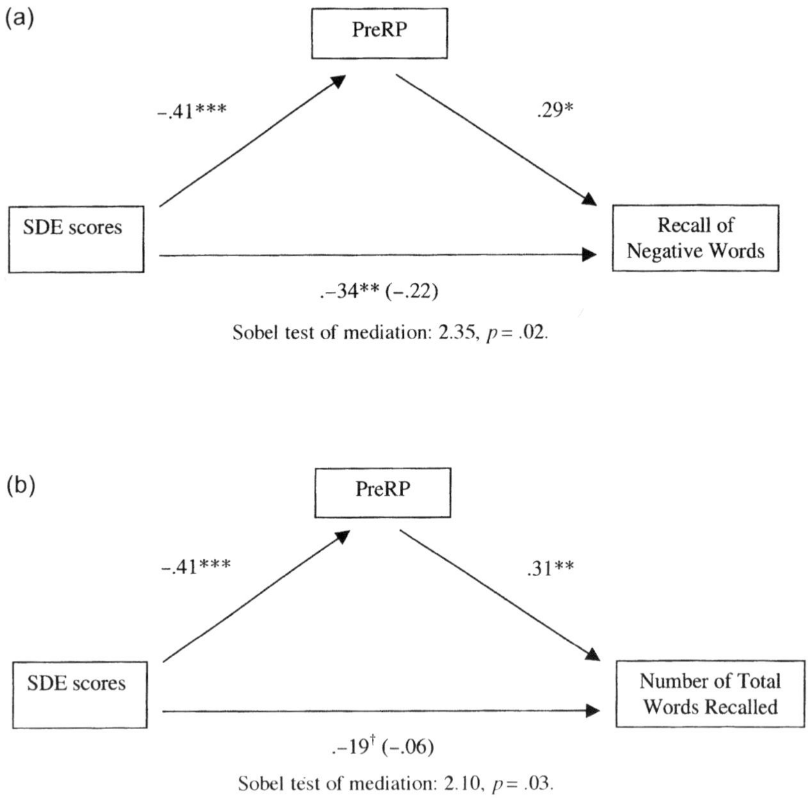

Figure 2. Mediation analyses to test the potential mediating effect of PreRP on the relationship between self-deceptive enhancement and memory for negative words.

of total words. A reduction in the correlation between SDE and memory distortions once PreRP was included in the model would indicate the predicted mediation. Figures 2a and 2b display the relationship in graphical form. As can be seen, in Figure 2a, PreRP did significantly mediate the relationship between SDE scores and reduced memory for negative words, as confirmed by a Sobel test of mediation (Baron & Kenny, 1986). A similar pattern is displayed in Figure 2b for total recall ability. Although SDE scores only tended toward initial predictive validity, the Sobel test of mediation again demonstrated a significant mediational influence of PreRP on the SDE-memory relationship. It appears, then, that repressors' decreased memory—at least for negatively valenced information—is mediated by their reduced allocation of processing resources toward the retrieval of previously encoded information. This model did not predict memory for positive or neutral words, providing further evidence in support of the notion that this reduced allocation is motivated by the exposure to negatively valenced or aversive information.

DISCUSSION

The present study sought to link the creation of self-induced memory distortions to decreased processing of negatively valenced information during the encoding and/or retrieval of such information. In support of this notion, lower levels of both PostRP and PreRP were significantly associated with reduced ability to recall negative words from a list including positive, negative, and neutral words. PostRP indexed the extent to which processing resources were allocated toward the encoding of negative information in relation to the encoding of equivalent positive information. PreRP, in contrast, indexed the extent to which processing resources were allocated toward the retrieval of previously experienced negative information, in relation to the retrieval of equivalent positive information. These results, therefore, demonstrate that a reduced allocation of processing resources during either the encoding or retrieval of negative information may cause diminished memorial capacity. Of particular import, level of PostRP and/or PreRP were not only predictive of the ability to recall negative words, but were also predictive of the recall of positive words, and of overall memory capacity. It may be, then, that a reduction in the processing of negative information is an indication of a generally inferior processing strategy, which causes global deficits in memory formation. Alternatively, it may be that negative feedback, indicating error in goal-directed behaviour (Peterson, 1999; Peterson & Flanders, 2002), may inherently hold a greater amount of potential information than positive feedback, indicating success (see Podsakoff & Farh, 1989; Talkington, Altman, & Grinnell, 1971; Wilson, Meyers, & Gilbert, 2001 for further evidence to suggest that negative information may hold more information). Under this conception, reduced processing of negatively valent information may simultaneously reduce the extent to which knowledge can be garnered from such information (see Shane & Peterson, in press, for direct evidence in support of this hypothesis).

The current study also sought to investigate the possibility that reduced levels of PostRP and/or PreRP may be responsible for the memory distortions characteristic of repressive individuals. A decreased level of PostRP in repressors would indicate avoidance of cognitive processing upon initial exposure to unwanted information. Conversely, a decreased level of PreRP in repressors would indicate processing restrictions employed during more elaborative processing, or upon re-exposure to the unwanted information, when automatically activated memory traces (Baddeley, 1999; Baddeley & Hitch, 1994) are triggered. Limited elaborative processing may create a less robust memory trace for the particular information, whereas reduced processing during the retrieval of negative information may directly limit the conscious recollection of that information, regardless of the strength of the particular memory trace.

The results of the present study indicated that individuals classified as repressors using a double median split of the SDE and the TMAS evidenced significantly reduced levels of PreRP, but not PostRP, compared to non-repressors. Thus, repressors were characterised by reduced levels of active processing during the retrieval, but not during the initial encoding, of negatively valenced information. This result is consistent with a subset of the current literature, which has found evidence for retrieval-based processing deficits in repressors (e.g., Holtgraves & Hall, 1995; Lorig et al., 1994), and suggests that the memorial distortions characteristic of repressive individuals may generally be due to a less thorough attempt to investigate negatively valenced retrieved memories. It should be noted that previous research has demonstrated reduced levels of PostRP in repressors, however, suggesting that reduced encoding may, at times, also play a role in repressors' memory distortions (Shane & Peterson, in press; see also Schimmack & Hartmann, 1997). It may be that repression can occur through either reduced encoding or reduced retrieval of unwanted information, and thus the reduced level of PreRP evidenced in the present repressor population may be identifying a different manifestation of a similar underlying construct.[3]

Another possibility, suggested by numerous researchers (e.g., Bjork, 1989; Bonanno et al., 1991; Hasher & Zacks, 1988; Myers et al., 1998), is that

[3] Shane and Peterson (in press) also utilised a slightly different go/no-go procedure than was employed in the present study. Primarily, two differences were evident. First, participant's received a monetary reward for each correct answer, and a monetary punishment for each incorrect answer, which may have increased the level of motivation of the participants (both to succeed, and to avoid the negative information). Second, the first five trials in Shane and Peterson (in press) included all 5 correct stimuli, which served to create a dominant ''go'' response. This 5-trial ''go pretreatment'' was not included in the present version of the task. Exactly how this may have influenced the results is unknown, however, Newman and colleagues (e.g., Newman & Kosson, 1986) have demonstrated that this ''go pretreatment'' is necessary to demonstrate significant deficits in certain populations.

repressors may show globally enhanced levels of inhibitory control, which better enable them to inhibit processing of unwanted information. Although consistent with the present notions regarding a reduction in the processing of aversive information, such theories suggest a purely cognitive explanation for repressor's memory distortions. In contrast, the present authors put forward a model which implicates motivated attempts to regulate affect, mood, and self-concept as additional influences regarding the formation of such memorial distortions. This notion is in line with previous theorisations that have posited emotive, mood-repair, or self-protective influences on memory distortions (e.g., Conway & Ross, 1984; Levine, 1997; McFarland & Alvaro, 2000; McFarland & Buehler, 1997, 1998; Ross & Wilson, 2002; Safer & Keuler, 2002; Wilson & Ross, 2001).

The results of the present study in fact provide evidence for both global memorial deficits, and specific strategic deficits for memory of aversive information. Repressors exhibited a pattern of reduced memory for negative, positive, and neutral words, in relation to nonrepressors, which culminated in a tendency toward a difference in overall memory performance between the two groups. This may represent a general memorial deficit in repressors, which would be consistent with research suggesting that high levels of cortisol may impair memory as a consequence of hippocampal damage (Pugh, Tremblay, Fleshner, & Rudy, 1997; Roozendaal, 2000). Shane and Peterson's (in press, 2004) have, additionally, suggested that reduced processing of negative information may cause broad-based cognitive and behavioural deficiencies due to subsequent and cumulative deficits in learning-predicated conception, skill and habit.

In addition to the evidence of global memory impairment, however, the present study indicated that repressors seem to have particular difficulty remembering negatively valent information. In fact, despite the observed trend toward a general reduction in recalled words, only repressor's memory of negative words showed a statistically significant deficit. A similar pattern of negative-specific memory weakness has been reported by Myers et al. (1998) with positive and negative words, and Bonanno et al. (1991), with aural presentation of threatening and nonthreatening information. Furthermore, repressors memory for negative autobiographical information has shown evidence of weakness as well (Davis, 1987; Davis & Schwartz, 1987). Thus, there is considerable evidence to suggest that repression may not be adequately explained by theories that posit the use of a generally enhanced inhibitory mechanism. Rather, it appears that repressors are particularly motivated to avoid processing negative information, and thus may strategically engage in more strenuous attempts to inhibit such information than nonrepressors. This additional effort undertaken during exposure to negative information, rather than an overproductive inhibitory mechanism, may then be responsible for repressors' memory distortions.

The present study also provides evidence to suggest that level of self-reported anxiety may not, in fact, be an important or accurate predictor of repressive personalities, or of memorial distortions. When continuous analyses were performed, using TMAS, SDE and TMAS × SDE as individual predictors of anxiety, only SDE showed any ability to predict the memorial and attentional performance of the participants in the present study. One possibility, then, is that anxiety is not a crucial predictor of these behaviours. This interpretation, if correct, would explain the existence of the "defensive high anxious" group, which has confused researchers to date with their seemingly unlikely combination of personality traits. Another possibility is that the SDE accounts for the same portion of the variance as anxiety normally would. Consistent with this notion, the SDE and TMAS were moderately correlated in the present sample. Zero order correlations between anxiety and memory performance did not reach significance, however. A third and final possibility is that the TMAS × SDE interaction may not provide easily interpretable data. Weinberger (1995) created the categorical distinctions used in the present study for just this reason: He posited that the advantage of a categorical analysis over multiple regression using two continuous dimensions is the potential to identify asymmetrical group patterns. In other words, traditional interaction terms would be most sensitive to disordinal "crossovers", yet it would be rare that opposite groups (e.g., low anxious vs. defensive high anxious individuals) behave in a similar manner (see also Mendolia, 2003, who has recently created the "index of self-regulation of emotion", which also avoids using regression analyses).

Taylor and Brown (1988) have suggested that the use of repressive-like processes are normal and healthy, and protect against anxiety and depressive disorders. The present findings confer with a number of additional findings that have recently suggested that there may be long-term deficits to a repressive strategy, despite the potential for short-term anxiety amelioration. Specifically, it appears that strategically reducing the extent to which negative information is processed has a significant effect on the extent to which that information can be recalled at a later time. Shane and Peterson (in press) have, in fact, even more directly demonstrated that the extent to which processing resources are allocated toward negative information influences the ability to learn from that information, and to utilise that information to effectively adapt previously dysfunctional action patterns. Thus, although individuals who utilise such motivated cognitive avoidance techniques may rate themselves as happier, and may evidence reduced levels of stress and anxiety after severe trauma, serious cognitive and intellectual effects may result, of which the entire implications remain somewhat unclear. Future research will, one hopes, continue to investigate this issue, to better determine the specific effects that such repressive tendencies can cause.

REFERENCES

Baddeley, A. D. (1999). *Essentials of human memory*. Hove, UK: Psychology Press.

Baddeley, A. D., & Hitch, G. J. (1994). Developments in the concept of working memory. *Neuropsychology, 8*, 485–493.

Bahrick, H. P., Hall, L. K., & Berger, S. A. (1996). Accuracy and distortion in memory for high school grades. *Psychological Science, 7*, 265–271.

Baron, R. M., & Kenny, D. A. (1986). The moderator-mediator variable distinction in social psychological research: Conceptual, strategic, and statistical considerations. *Journal of Personality and Social Psychology, 51*, 1173–1182.

Bjork, R. A. (1989). Retrieval inhibition as an adaptive mechanism in human memory. In Roediger, H. L. III & Craik, F. I. M. (Eds.), *Varieties of memory and consciousness: Essays in honour of Endel Tulving*. (pp. 309–330). Hillsdale, NJ: Erlbaum.

Boden, J. M., & Baumeister, R. F. (1997). Repressive coping: Distraction using pleasant thoughts and memories. *Journal of Personality and Social Psychology, 73*, 45–62.

Bonanno, G. A., Davis, P. J., Singer, J. L., & Schwartz, G. E. (1991). The repressor personality and avoidant information processing: A dichotic listening study. *Journal of Research in Personality, 25*, 386–401.

Bower, G. H. (1981). Mood and memory. *American Psychologist, 36*, 129–148.

Brewin, C. R. (2001). Memory processes in post-traumatic stress disorder. *International Review of Psychiatry, 13*, 159–163.

Brosschot, J. F., De Ruiter, C., & Kindt, M. (1999). Recall and recognition of threatening, pleasant, and neutral words in repressors. *European Journal of Personality, 13*, 1–14.

Brown, L. T., Tomarken, A. J., Orth, D. N, Loosen, P. T., Kalin, N. H., & Davidson, R. J. (1996). Individual differences in repressive-defensiveness predict basal salivary cortisol levels. *Journal of Personality and Social Psychology, 70*, 362–371.

Conway, M., & Ross, M. (1984). Getting what you want by revising what you had. *Journal of Personality and Social Psychology, 47*, 738–748.

Crowne, D. P., & Marlow, D. (1960). A new scale of social desirability independent of psychopathology. *Journal of Consulting Psychology, 24*, 349–354.

Damasio, A. (1994). *Descartes' error: Emotion, reason, and the human brain*. New York: Putnam.

Davis, P. J. (1987). Repression and the inaccessibility of affective memories. *Journal of Personality and Social Psychology, 53*, 585–593.

Davis, P. J., & Schwartz, G. E. (1987). Repression and the inaccessibility of affective memories. *Journal of Personality and Social Psychology, 52*, 155–162.

Dawkins, K., & Furnham, A. (1989). The colour naming of emotional words. *British Journal of Psychology, 80*, 383–389.

Feldman-Summers, S., & Pope, K. S. (1994). The experience of "forgetting" childhood abuse: A national survey of psychologists. *Journal of Consulting and Clinical Psychology, 62*, 636–639.

Foa, E. B., Molnar, C., & Cashman, L. (1995). Change in rape narratives during exposure therapy for posttraumatic stress disorder [Special Issue]. *Journal of Traumatic Stress, 8*, 675–690.

Fox, E. (1993). Allocation of visual attention and anxiety. *Cognition and Emotion, 7*, 207–215.

Freud, S. (1957). On the history of the psychoanalytic movement, papers on metapsychology, and other works. In J. Strachey (Ed. & Trans.), *The collected works of Sigmund Freud* (Vol. 14). New York: Basic Books. (Original work published 1901)

Fuller, B. F. (1992). The effects of stress-anxiety and coping styles on heart rate variability. *International Journal of Psychophysiology, 12*, 81–86.

Furnham, A., Petrides, K. V., & Spencer-Bowdage, S. (2002). The effects of different types of social desirability on the identification of repressors. *Personality and Individual Differences, 33*, 119–130.

Hansen, R. D., & Hansen, C. H. (1988). Repression of emotionally tagged memories: The architecture of less complex emotions. *Journal of Personality and Social Psychology*, *55*, 811–818.

Hansen, C. H., Hansen, R. D., & Shantz, D. W. (1992). Repression at encoding: Discrete appraisals of emotional stimuli. *Journal of Personality and Social Psychology*, *63*, 1026–1035.

Harvey, A. G., & Bryant, R. A. (1999). The relationship between acute stress disorder and posttraumatic stress disorder A 2-year prospective evaluation. *Journal of Consulting and Clinical Psychology*, *67*, 985–988.

Hasher, L., & Zacks, R. T. (1988). Working memory, comprehension, and aging: A review and a new view. In Bower, G. H. (Ed.), *The psychology of learning and motivation: Advances in research and theory* (Vol. 22, pp. 193–225). San Diego, CA: Academic Press.

Hock, M., Krohne, H. W., & Kaiser, J. (1996). Coping dispositions and the processing of ambiguous stimuli. *Journal of Personality and Social Psychology*, *70*, 1052–1066.

Holtgraves, T., & Hall, R. (1995). Repressors: What do they repress and how do they repress it? *Journal of Research in Personality*, *29*, 306–317.

Jamner, L. D., Schwartz, G. E., & Leigh, H. (1988). The relationship between repressive and defensive coping stylesand monocyte, eosinophile, and serum glucose levels: Support for the opiod peptide hypothesis of repression. *Psychosomatic Medicine*, *50*, 567–575.

Kučera, H., & Francis, W. N. (1967). *Computational analysis of present day American English*. Providence, RI: Brown University Press.

Lane, R. D., Schwartz, G. E. (1987). Induction of lateralized sympathetic input to the heart by the CNS during emotional arousal: A possible neurophysiologic trigger of sudden cardiac death. *Psychosomatic Medicine*, *49*, 274–284.

Levine, L. J. (1997). Reconstructing memory for emotions. *Journal of Experimental Psychology. General*, *126*, 165–177.

Loftus, E. F., Polansky, S., & Fullilove, M. T. (1994). Memories of childhood sexual abuse: Remembering and repressing. *Psychology of Women Quarterly*, *18*, 67–84.

Lorig, T. S., Singer, J. L., Bonanno, G. A., Davis, P. & Schwartz, G. (1994). Repressor personality styles and EEG patterns associated with affective memory and thought suppression. *Imagination, Cognition and Personality*, *14*, 203–210.

Mazzoni, G. (2002). Naturally occurring and suggestion-dependent memory distortions: The convergence of disparate research traditions. *European Psychologist*, *7*, 17–30.

McDonald, H. E., & Hirt, E. R. (1997). When expectancy meets desire: Motivational effects in reconstructive memory. *Journal of Personality and Social Psychology*, *72*, 5–23.

McFarland, C., & Alvaro, C. (2000). The impact of motivation on temporal comparisons: Coping with traumatic events by perceiving personal growth. *Journal of Personality and Social Psychology*, *79*, 327–343.

McFarland, C., & Buehler, R. (1997). Negative affective states and the motivated retrival of positive life events: the role of affect acknowledgment. *Journal of Personality and Social Psychology*, *73*, 200–214.

McFarland, C., & Buehler, R. (1998). The impact of negative affect on autobiographical memory: The role of self-focused attention to moods. *Journal of Personality and Social Psychology*, *75*, 1424–1440.

Mendolia, M. (2003). An index of self-regulation of emotion and the study of repression in social contexts that threaten or do not threaten self-concept. *Emotion*, *2*, 215–232.

Myers, L. B., & Brewin, C. R. (1995). Repressive coping and the recall of emotional material. *Cognition and Emotion*, *9*, 637–642.

Myers, L. B., Brewin, C. R., & Power, M. J. (1998). Repressive coping and the directed forgetting of emotional material. *Journal of Abnormal Psychology*, *107*, 141–148.

Newman, L. S., & Hedberg, D. A. (1999). Repressive coping and the inaccessibility of negative autobiographical memories: Converging evidence. *Personality and Individual Differences*, *27*, 45–53.

Newman, J. P., Patterson, C. M., Howland, E. W., & Nichols, S. L. (1990). Passive avoidance in psychopaths: The effects of reward. *Personality and Individual Differences*, *11*, 1101–1114.

Oldenburg, C., & Kivistoe, P. (2002). Explicit and implicit memory, trait anxiety, and repressive coping style. *Personality and Individual Differences*, *32*, 107–119.

Paulhus, D. L. (1991). Measurement and control of response bias. In Robinson, J. P., Shaver, P. R., et al. (Eds.), *Measures of personality and social psychological attitudes* (Vol. 1, pp. 17–59). San Diego, CA: Academic Press.

Paulhus, D. L., & John, O. P. (1998). Egoistic and moralistic biases in self-perception: The interplay of self-deceptive styles with basic traits and motives [Special Issue]. *Journal of Personality*, *66*, 1025–1060.

Peterson, J. B. (1999). *Maps of meaning: The architecture of belief.* Florence, KY: Taylor & Francis.

Peterson, J. B., & Flanders, J. L. (2002). Complexity management theory: Motivation for ideological rigidity and social conflict. *Cortex*, *38*, 429–458.

Podsakoff, P. M., & Farh, J. (1989). Effects of feedback sign and credibility on goal setting and task performance. *Organizational Behavior and Human Decision Processes*, *44*, 45–67.

Pugh, C. R., Tremblay, D., Fleshner, M., & Rudy, J. W. (1997). A selective role for corticosterone in contextual-fear conditioning. *Behavioral Neuroscience*, *111*, 503–511.

Roozendaal, B. (2000). Glucocoritocoids and the regulation of memory consolidation. *Psychoneuroendocrinology*, *25*, 213–238.

Ross, M., & Wilson, A. E. (2002). It feels like yesterday: Self-esteem, valence of personal past experiences, and judgments of subjective distance. *Journal of Personality and Social Psychology*, *82*, 792–803.

Safer, M. A., & Keuler, D. J. (2002). Individual differences in misremembering pre-psychotherapy distress: Personality and memory distortion. *Emotion*, *2*, 162–178.

Shafrir, U., & Pascual-Leone, J. (1990). Postfailure reflectivity/impulsivity and spontaneous attention to errors. *Journal of Educational Psychology*, *82*, 378–387.

Shane, M. S., & Peterson, J. B. (in press). Self-deceivers show increased passive-avoidance errors on Newman's go/nogo task: Implications for self-deception and socialization. *Journal of Personality*.

Shane, M. S., & Peterson, J. B. (2004). *Reflective preference predicts learning over and above IQ: It isn't the size (of your intellect) that matters, but how you use it.* Manuscript under review.

Schimmack, U., & Hartmann, K. (1997). Individual differences in the memory representation of emotional episodes: Exploring the cognitive processes in repression. *Journal of Personality and Social Psychology*, *73*, 1064–1079.

Talkington, L. W., Altman, R., & Grinnell, T. K. (1971). Effects of positive and negative feedback on the motor performance of mongoloids. *Perceptual and Motor Skills*, *33*, 1075–1078.

Taylor, J. A. (1953). A personality scale of manifest anxiety. *Journal of Abnormal and Social Psychology*, *48*, 285–290.

Taylor, S. E., & Brown, J. D. (1988). Illusion and well-being: A social psychological perspective on mental health. *Psychological Bulletin*, *103*, 193–210.

Tromp, S., Koss, M. P., Figueredo, A. J., & Tharan, M. (1995). Are rape memories different? A comparison of rape, other unpleasant and pleasant memories among employed women [Special Issue]. *Journal of Traumatic Stress*, *8*, 607–627.

Weinberger, D. A. (1995). The construct validity of the repressive coping style. In J. L. Singer (Ed), *Repression and dissociation: Implications for personality theory, psychopathology, and health* (pp. 337–386). Chicago: University of Chicago Press.

Weinberger, D. A., Schwartz, G. E, & Davidson, R. J. (1979). Low-anxious, high-anxious, and repressive coping styles: Psychometric patterns and behavioral and physiological responses to stress. *Journal of Abnormal Psychology*, *88*, 369–380.

Williams, L. M. (1994). Recall of childhood trauma: A prospective study of women's memories of child sexual abuse. *Journal of Consulting and Clinical Psychology*, *62*, 1167–1176.

Wilson, T. D., Meyers, J., & Gilbert, D. T. (2001). Lessons from the past: Do people learn from experience that emotional reactions are short-lived? *Personality and Social Psychology Bulletin*, *27*, 1648–1661.

Wilson, A. E., & Ross, M. (2001). From chump to champ: People's appraisals of their earlier and present selves. *Journal of Personality and Social Psychology*, *80*, 572–584.

Wright, D. B. (2003). Making friends with your data: Improving how statistics are reported and conducted. *British Journal of Educational Psychology*, *73*, 123–136.

COGNITION AND EMOTION, 2004, *18* (4), 559–574

Painting with broad strokes: Happiness and the malleability of event memory

Linda J. Levine
University of California, Irvine, USA

Susan Bluck
University of Florida, Gainesville, USA

Individuals often feel that they remember positive events better than negative ones, but do they? To investigate the relation between emotional valence and the malleability of memory for real-world events, we assessed participants' emotions and memories concerning the televised announcement of the verdict in the murder trial of O. J. Simpson. Memory was assessed for actual events and plausible foils. Participants who were happy about the verdict reported recalling events with greater clarity after two months, and recognised more events after a year, than participants whose reaction to the verdict was negative, irrespective of whether the events had occurred or not. Signal detection analyses confirmed that the threshold for judging events as having occurred was lower for participants who were happy about the verdict. These findings demonstrate that the association between happiness and reconstructive memory errors, previously shown in laboratory studies, extends to memory for real-world events and over prolonged time periods.

Research on autobiographical memory has shown that, in general, positive life events are remembered slightly better than negative life events (Walker, Skowronski, & Thompson, 2003). For example, Walker, Vogl, and Thompson (1997) had participants keep diaries for three months and rate the pleasantness or unpleasantness of recorded events. At the end of the three months, participants again rated the events for pleasantness and also rated how well they remembered them. The results showed that pleasant events were remembered better than unpleasant events. The degree of pleasantness associated with events, both initially and at the time of retrieval, predicted participants' memory clarity ratings. A closer look at this literature though shows a puzzling finding. When

Correspondence should be addressed to Linda J. Levine, Department of Psychology and Social Behavior, University of California, Irvine, 3340 Social Ecology II, Irvine, California 92697-7085, USA; e-mail: llevine@uci.edu

We thank Susan Charles, Heather Lench, and Martin Safer for comments on previous drafts.

http://www.tandf.co.uk/journals/pp/02699931.html DOI:10.1080/02699930341000446

people are asked to make subjective memory judgements, they typically indicate that events that evoked positive emotion are more clearly remembered (e.g., Matlin & Stang, 1978; Thompson, Skowronski, Larsen, & Betz, 1996; Walker et al., 1997), or come to mind more quickly (Master, Lishman, & Smith, 1983), than events that evoked negative emotion. When researchers look at the objective accuracy of people's accounts, however, they sometimes find no valence effect (e.g., Holmes, 1970), or superior memory for negative events (e.g., Banaji & Hardin, 1994; Bluck & Li, 2001; Kreitler & Kreitler, 1968). Thus, it appears that people may believe they remember happy events more clearly than they really do.

One explanation for these conflicting findings is suggested by recent work on the differing information-processing strategies associated with positive and negative emotion. Researchers have argued that people feel happy when goals are achieved and there is no immediate problem to be solved. Because general knowledge is typically adequate for maintaining a state of well-being in such circumstances, people tend to draw freely on general knowledge when they feel happy. In contrast, negative emotions are experienced when goals are threatened or have failed. People in a negative mood tend to engage in effortful processing, evaluating information in a careful, systematic manner and relying less on general knowledge and heuristics. Thus emotional valence, which reflects whether or not there is a problem to be solved, is thought to influence people's information-processing strategies (for a review see Bless & Schwarz, 1999).

A growing body of laboratory research in social psychology is consistent with this view. In several studies, people have been put in a positive or negative mood and then asked to evaluate the strength of arguments. The results indicate that happy people are influenced more by prior beliefs or heuristics (such as the belief that experts produce better arguments than novices) than are people in neutral or sad moods who in turn attend more to the specific content of arguments to evaluate their quality (e.g., Bless, Bohner, Schwarz, & Strack, 1990; Mackie & Worth, 1989). Similarly, when asked to judge other people's culpability or personality attributes, happy people rely more on general knowledge (Fiedler, Asbeck, & Nickle, 1991), stereotypes (Bodenhausen, Kramer, & Susser, 1994), or heuristics (Forgas, 2002) than do people in a neutral or negative mood. Happiness also has been shown to facilitate flexibility and creativity in categorisation and other problem-solving tasks (e.g., Fredrickson, 2001; Isen, Daubman, & Nowicki, 1987). In contrast, people in negative moods tend to process information in a data-driven manner and are more conservative in their judgements.

Recent findings indicate that the differing information processing strategies associated with positive and negative emotion also affect memory. For example, Bless and his colleagues induced a happy or sad mood in participants, and then presented them with information about common activities such as eating at a restaurant (Bless et al., 1996). Some of the information was script typical (e.g., "the hostess placed the menus on the table"), and some was script atypical (e.g., "he put away his tennis racket"). Participants were later given a surprise recognition test that included both previously presented and new information. They found that happy participants were more likely than sad participants to "recognise" script typical information, independent of whether or not the information had actually been presented. Sad participants were more conservative, and more accurate, in their recognition judgements. Park and Banaji (2000) found that happy participants showed a bias toward greater leniency in recognising ethnic names as members of stereotypical categories, leading to many instances of false recognition. In contrast, participants in a negative mood used a more stringent criterion when making recognition judgements. Thus, happiness can lead to greater reliance on general knowledge or stereotypes, and to intrusion errors, in memory.

These effects have been demonstrated in the laboratory using short-term induced moods and experimental stimuli, but little if any research has examined the relation of happiness to reconstructive memory errors in the real world. Much of the research on memory failures has examined memory for neutral stimuli (for a review see Koriat, Goldsmith, & Pansky, 2000) or for traumatic events that evoked intense negative emotions (e.g., Yuille & Tollestrup, 1992). Although the literature has gained greatly from those investigations, our goal in the current study was to find out if people make reconstructive errors when they recall real-world events that made them happy. We hypothesised that, when recalling happy events, people may "paint with broad strokes", drawing on information encoded when events first occurred but also drawing freely on their general knowledge about what is plausible to fill in gaps in their representations. If so, we would expect happy memories to be associated with greater subjective memory clarity, but also with more intrusion errors, than negative memories.

To test this hypothesis, we assessed memory for both true, and plausible but false, details of a real world event that could be verified objectively. To minimise differences between negative and positive events unrelated to emotion, we examined memory for a single event that evoked positive emotion in some people and negative emotion in others.

The present investigation

On 3 October 1995, Orenthal James (O. J.) Simpson was acquitted of the murders of his former wife, Nicole Brown Simpson, and her friend, Ron Goldman. The announcement of the verdict was televised live in the United States with all stations airing the same coverage of the courtroom proceedings. The verdict was of intense interest to many Americans because the defendant was a former football hero and because the trial raised thorny issues about equity between races in the American criminal justice system and about spousal abuse. We assessed the emotions and memories of individuals who first found out the verdict by watching the live announcement on television. Participants completed questionnaires one week, two months, and an average of 14 months after the verdict was announced. At each time point, they described how they felt, both when they first learned of the verdict, and when they thought about the verdict now. After two months, participants rated how clearly they recalled events in the courtroom that immediately followed the verdict announcement. After 14 months, participants were given a recognition test in which they indicated whether or not they remembered each event and rated their confidence in their answers.

The objectives of the study were: (a) to examine the relation between the emotional valence of an event and people's *subjective* judgement of the clarity with which they remember the event; (b) to examine the relation between valence and *objective* memory accuracy; (c) to explore whether emotional valence at the time of encoding or retrieval better predicts memory clarity and accuracy; and (d) to assess whether the association between happiness and reconstructive errors, previously demonstrated in brief laboratory studies using stimuli such as simple narratives and lists of names, generalises to events and to periods of time that are ecologically relevant to everyday memory and autobiographical memory.

We predicted that feeling happy about the verdict would be associated with greater subjective memory clarity, but more reconstructive memory errors, than feeling negative about the verdict. When asked whether they remember an event, people may subject their recollected experience to careful scrutiny, resulting in conservative judgements. Alternatively, they may draw flexibly on general knowledge about what might have occurred as well as on experience at the time of encoding, resulting in more liberal judgements. Signal detection analyses were conducted to test the prediction that people use a more liberal criterion for judging that they remember events, when the events in question evoked positive as opposed to negative emotion.

METHOD

Design and procedure

The study used a quasi-experimental design with repeated measures. Participants completed questionnaires seven days, two months, and more than a year after the announcement of the verdict in the criminal trial of O. J. Simpson. The first questionnaire assessed participants' initial emotional reactions to the verdict announcement, desired verdict, memory performance predictors (prior knowledge, rehearsal), and demographic information. The second and third questionnaires assessed participants' current feelings about the verdict and memory for details of the verdict announcement.

This study was part of a larger project that also examined people's memory for their past emotions (Levine & Bluck, in press; Levine, Prohaska, Burgess, Rice, & Laulhere, 2001). The current paper presents original findings concerning memory for emotional events. In this study, only participants who watched the initial televised announcement of the verdict were included.

Participants

Time 1. Seven days after the verdict was announced, questionnaires were completed by 156 undergraduates in a psychology class at the University of California, Irvine: 69% of the participants were female. The ethnicities of the participants approximated the demographics of the campus; they were Asian (42%), Hispanic (28%), Caucasian (24%), African American (2%), and other (4%). Participants ranged in age from 17 to 34 years ($M = 19$, $SD = 1.93$).

Time 2. Two months (56 days) after the verdict was announced, a second questionnaire was completed by 139 of the initial participants. Preliminary analyses revealed no significant differences between students who completed the second questionnaire and students who did not, in terms of demographics, initial emotions, desired verdict, prior knowledge about the verdict or rehearsal.

Time 3. A third questionnaire was completed by 87 of the initial participants over a year after the verdict was announced (M = 14 months, range = 12–16 months). No significant differences were found on demographic, emotion or memory variables when comparing students who completed the third questionnaire and students who did not, with the exception that more females (77%) than males (23%) responded to the third questionnaire.

To avoid anticipatory rehearsal, participants were not informed that they would be questioned again concerning the verdict before receiving the second and third questionnaires. Participants received course credit for completing the first two questionnaires and five dollars for completing the third questionnaire.

Questionnaires

Time 1. The initial questionnaire assessed participants' emotions with the question, "When you first learned of the verdict, how intensely did you feel each emotion listed below?" Participants rated how happy, angry, and sad they felt using 5-point scales ranging from 0 (*not at all*) to 4 (*extremely*). Participants also indicated what verdict they desired (*not guilty, guilty, did not care*). As a measure of prior knowledge about the trial, participants were asked to estimate how much time they had spent each week, in the month before the verdict was announced, watching TV, reading newspapers, or listening to radio accounts concerning the trial. Rehearsal was assessed by asking participants to estimate how much time they had spent, since the verdict was announced, thinking or talking about what went on in the courtroom when the verdict was announced. Prior knowledge and rehearsal were rated on 5-point scales (*none*; *1–3 hours*; *4–6 hours*; *7–9 hours*; *more than 9 hours*).

Time 2. After two months, participants used 5-point scales to rate how happy, angry, and sad they felt when they thought about the verdict now. Participants also rated the clarity with which they recalled ten events concerning the verdict announcement on a scale ranging from 0 (*not at all clearly*) to 4 (*very clearly*). Half of these events had actually occurred, for example: "O. J. Simpson mouthed the words 'thank you' to the jury", "Johnny Cochran (defence lawyer) pressed his face against Mr Simpson's shoulder". Half were plausible but had not occurred, for example: "O. J. Simpson gave the 'thumb's up' sign to his lawyer, Robert Shapiro", "Judge Ito told audience members they would have to leave if there were any further disruptions". Both the true and false events were chosen to represent all the major "players" in the verdict announcement. This was done to avoid the possibility that individuals who focused differentially on either the prosecution or defense side would be advantaged in memory performance.

Time 3. The questionnaire administered after more than a year was identical to the questionnaire administered after 2 months, with two exceptions. First, memory was assessed for an additional 10 events of the verdict announcement, so that in total, participants rated their memory for 20 events. As in the second questionnaire, half of the events had occurred and half were plausible but had not occurred.[1] Second, memory questions after a year were framed to distinguish between accuracy and confidence. Thus, instead of rating the clarity with which they recalled each event, participants first indicated whether or not they recalled the event (*yes, no*) and then rated how sure they were that they were correct on a scale ranging from 0 (*not at all sure*) to 4 (*very sure*). Final course grades for participants were also obtained.

RESULTS

Initially-reported emotions and desired verdict

What were participants' initial reactions to Simpson's acquittal? A week after the verdict, 27% of the participants reported that they desired a verdict of not guilty; 49% desired a verdict of guilty; and 24% did not care. Participants' initial emotional reactions to the verdict were expected to vary depending on

[1] To find out if false events were as plausible as true events, we presented the 10 true and 10 false events to two (previously untested) groups of undergraduates 14 months after the verdict had been announced. One group had viewed the verdict announcement on TV ($n = 47$); the other group had not ($n = 53$). Participants were asked to indicate whether or not they thought each event had occurred. If false events were not as plausible as true events, then the "No TV" group should have endorsed more true than false items. No significant difference was found, however, in the number of true ($M = 4.77$) and false events ($M = 4.94$) endorsed by the No TV group, $t = -0.51$, n.s. In contrast, the group that had viewed the events on TV endorsed more true events ($M = 5.14$) than false events ($M = 4.32$), $t = 2.97$, $p = .01$.

the verdict they desired. To confirm this, and to check for differences related to gender and ethnicity, we conducted a MANOVA on participants' initial intensity ratings for happiness, anger, and sadness. The between-subject variables were desired verdict, gender, and ethnicity. As anticipated, an interaction was found between desired verdict and emotion, $F(4, 296) = 80.46$, $MS_e = 0.97$, $p < .0001$. No other significant interactions with emotion were found. Table 1 shows mean initial intensity ratings, and significant contrasts, for happiness, anger, and sadness by desired verdict. These findings simply demonstrate that the verdict announcement was a happy or positive event for participants who desired a verdict of not guilty, a negative event for participants who desired a verdict of guilty, and a relatively neutral event for participants who did not care. Therefore, we analysed memory variables by the desired verdict (not guilty, guilty, did not care) to see if the verdict announcement was remembered differently by participants whose reaction to the verdict was positive, negative or neutral.

Before assessing memory, preliminary analyses were conducted to find out whether these three groups differed on variables likely to be related to memory: prior knowledge about the trial, rehearsal, and course grade (a measure of academic performance). These analyses included all participants who completed memory questions after 2 months ($N = 139$). ANOVAs, with desired verdict as the independent variable, showed no significant differences between groups with respect to rehearsal or course grade. Participants who did not care about the verdict, however, reported having less prior knowledge about the trial ($M = 0.69$, $SD = 0.62$) than either the positive group ($M = 1.09$, $SD = 0.71$) or the negative group ($M = 0.97$, $SD = 0.69$), who did not differ significantly from each other, $F(2, 136) = 3.23$, $MS_e = 1.48$, $p = .04$; critical value of $t(136) = 1.98$, $MS_e = 0.46$, $p < .05$. Analyses including all participants who completed memory questions after more than a year ($N = 87$) showed the identical pattern of results.

TABLE 1
Mean initial intensity ratings (and standard deviations) for happiness, anger, and sadness by desired verdict

Desired verdict	*n*	*Happiness*	*Anger*	*Sadness*
1. Not guilty	41	2.71 (1.19)	0.37 (0.80)	0.56 (0.71)
2. Guilty	76	0.26 (0.74)	2.64 (1.27)	2.46 (1.19)
3. Did not care	39	1.13 (1.08)	0.56 (0.64)	0.74 (0.99)
Contrasts		1 > 2 & 3; 3 > 2	2 > 1 & 3	2 > 1 & 3

Note: Post-hoc comparisons shown in the "Contrasts" row were conducted using Scheffé's F with a critical value of 3.06, $p < .05$, $MS_e = 0.80$ for happiness, 1.07 for anger, and 1.09 for sadness.

Memory clarity ratings after two months

Event valence and memory. After 2 months, participants rated how clearly they recalled 10 events, half true and half false. A MANCOVA (controlling for prior knowledge and rehearsal) was conducted with memory clarity ratings for true events and false events as the dependent variables. The independent variable was whether participants' reaction to the verdict was positive (i.e., desired acquittal), negative (i.e., desired conviction), or neutral (i.e., did not care).[2] Part A of Table 2 shows the mean memory clarity ratings for true and false events for the three groups. As would be expected, participants recalled events that had occurred ($M = 3.23$, $SD = 1.06$) more clearly than events that had not occurred ($M = 2.45$, $SD = 1.00$), $F(1, 134) = 16.50$, $MS_e = 0.58$, $p < .0001$. Participants who were happy about the verdict, however, recalled events more clearly ($M = 3.17$, $SD = 0.85$) than participants whose reaction was negative ($M = 2.79$, $SD = 0.82$) or neutral ($M = 2.63$, $SD = 0.95$), irrespective of whether the events had occurred or not, $F(2, 134) = 3.07$, $MS_e = 1.39$, $p = .05$; critical value of $t(134) = 1.98$, $MS_e = 0.70$, $p < .05$. No significant difference in memory clarity was found between participants whose reaction to the verdict was negative versus neutral. Rehearsal was also found to be positively associated with memory clarity ratings, $F(1, 134) = 6.65$, $MS_e = 1.39$, $p = .01$.

Further inspection of the mean clarity ratings for individual events showed that participants whose reaction to the verdict was positive rated the clarity of their memory as higher than participants whose reaction was either negative or

TABLE 2
Memory for true and false events for participants whose reaction to the verdict was positive, negative or neutral

		True events		*False events*	
Reaction to verdict	*n*	*M*	*(SD)*	*M*	*(SD)*
A. Mean memory clarity ratings after 2 months					
Positive	34	3.44	(0.18)	2.85	(0.16)
Negative	69	3.18	(0.12)	2.37	(0.11)
Neutral	36	3.13	(0.18)	2.23	(0.16)
B. Mean number of events recognised after 14 months					
Positive	20	6.19	(0.50)	5.54	(0.59)
Negative	48	4.89	(0.31)	3.84	(0.37)
Neutral	19	5.54	(0.51)	4.14	(0.60)

[2] The analyses of memory reported in this paper also were conducted including ethnicity and gender. Including these variables did not alter the significance of the emotional valence effects in any analysis.

neutral for 9 out of the 10 events. Thus, participants who were happy about the verdict reported recalling events with greater clarity, independent of whether or not the events had occurred.

Emotional intensity and memory. The next analysis was conducted to find out if the intensity of happiness predicted memory clarity, and, if so, whether initially reported happiness or happiness about the verdict at the time of retrieval better predicted memory clarity. A three-step hierarchical regression analysis was conducted predicting mean memory clarity ratings after two months. On the first step, we entered prior knowledge and rehearsal (5-point scales). On the second step, we entered participants' initial ratings of how happy, angry, and sad they felt about the verdict (5-point scales). On the third step, we entered participants' ratings of how happy, angry, and sad they felt about the verdict at the time of retrieval (5-point scales). The results are shown in Table 3. After controlling for the other variables (i.e., on Step 3 of the analysis), the happier participants felt about the verdict at the time of retrieval, the more clearly they reported remembering events, $t(138) = 3.06, p = .003$, ß = .29. Note that initially reported happiness was significant at Step 2, and also tended to predict memory clarity

TABLE 3
Summary of hierarchical regression analysis for variables predicting mean memory clarity ratings after 2 months ($N = 139$)

	Variable	*B*	*SE B*	*ß*
Step 1	Prior knowledge	.22	.10	.17*
	Rehearsal	.21	.08	.20*
Step 2	Prior knowledge	.17	.10	.13
	Rehearsal	.17	.08	.17*
	Initial happiness	.22	.06	.35***
	Initial anger	.07	.07	.13
	Initial sadness	.08	.07	.12
Step 3	Prior knowledge	.11	.10	.09
	Rehearsal	.15	.08	.15
	Initial happiness	.13	.07	.20
	Initial anger	.03	.08	.04
	Initial sadness	.07	.07	.11
	Current happiness	.26	.09	.29**
	Current anger	.10	.10	.15
	Current sadness	−.01	.08	−.02

Note: $R^2 = .09$ for Step 1; $\Delta R^2 = .08$ for Step 2; $\Delta R^2 = .05$ for Step 3 (*ps* < .05). *$p < .05$; **$p < .01$; ***$p < .001$.

B = unstandardised regression coefficient; *SE B* = standard error of *B*.

after other variables were entered into the model (i.e., on Step 3), but this finding did not reach conventional levels of significance, $t(138) = 1.88$, $p = .063$, ß = .20.

Recognition memory after a year

Event valence and memory. Participants' recognition judgements after more than a year were examined next. A MANCOVA (controlling for prior knowledge and rehearsal) was conducted on the number of true and false events recognised by participants whose emotional reaction to the verdict was positive, negative, or neutral. The results, which are displayed in part B of Table 2, showed a significant effect of valence, $F(2, 82) = 3.43$, $MS_e = 8.61$, $p = .04$. Participants who were happy about the verdict recognised more events ($M = 11.73$, $SD = 3.59$) than did participants whose reaction was negative ($M = 8.74$, $SD = 4.12$), irrespective of whether the events had occurred or not. Participants whose reaction was neutral did not differ in the number of events recognised from the positive or negative groups ($M = 9.68$, $SD = 4.64$); critical value of $t(82) = 1.99$, $MS_e = 4.65$, $p < .05$.[3] No other significant differences were found. An ANCOVA, controlling for prior knowledge and rehearsal, was also conducted on the total number of *correct* recognition responses given. The results showed no significant differences for participants whose emotional reaction to the verdict was positive ($M = 10.65$, $SD = 2.28$), negative ($M = 11.06$, $SD = 2.25$), or neutral ($M = 11.36$, $SD = 2.29$), $F(2, 82) = 0.49$, $MS_e = 2.28$, n.s.

Emotional valence and recognition judgement threshold. Participants who were happy about the verdict recognised more events after a year than participants who felt negative. We conducted signal detection analyses to find out if participants who were happy about the verdict were simply less able to discriminate between actual and plausible events (discriminability) or if they adopted a more liberal criterion for judging events as remembered (bias). We first obtained the hit rate (proportion of true events recognised) and false alarm rate (proportion of false events recognised). Because some participants had hit or false alarm rates of 0 or 1, a standard correction was applied to these rates so that measures of discriminability and bias could be calculated (Snodgrass & Corwin, 1988). Discrimination (D_L) and bias (C_L) indices were then calculated on log transformed data to allow a better approximation to a normal distribution.

[3] As Table 2 shows, the neutral group fell slightly below the negative group on memory clarity ratings, but fell between the positive and negative groups on the number of events recognised. Subjective assessments such as event importance, which may contribute to memory clarity judgements, tend to be positively correlated with emotional intensity (Thompson et al., 1996). Thus, people who feel neutral about events typically rate memory clarity as relatively low. Recognition judgements are better for teasing apart whether an event is remembered from other assessments such as importance. The key finding, however, was that the positive and negative groups differed significantly on both memory measures. The familiarity of events, tapped by both memory measures, was greater for participants whose reaction to the verdict was positive.

For the measure of discriminability (D_L), larger values indicate greater ability to discriminate events that occurred from those that did not occur. For the measure of response bias (C_L), a value less than 0 indicates a liberal response bias or tendency to judge events as having occurred; a value greater than 0 indicates a conservative response bias or a tendency to judge events as not having occurred.

Table 4 shows the mean hit and false alarm rates, and measures of discriminability and bias, for participants whose initial emotional reaction to the verdict was positive, negative, or neutral. Single-factor ANOVAs indicated that the groups did not differ significantly on the measure of discriminability (D_L), $F(2, 84) = 0.50$, $MS_e = 1.05$, n.s., but did differ on the measure of bias (C_L), $F(2, 84) = 3.42$, $MS_e = 0.99$, $p = .04$. Post-hoc analyses showed that participants who were happy about the verdict used a more liberal criterion for judging that events had occurred (Mean $C_L = -0.35$), whereas participants who reacted negatively used a more conservative criterion (Mean $C_L = 0.34$); critical value of Scheffé's $F(84) = 3.11$, $MS_e = 0.98$, $p < .05$. Participants whose reaction to the verdict was neutral did not differ significantly from the positive or negative groups (Mean $C_L = 0.17$).

Emotional intensity and memory. We conducted a hierarchical regression analysis to explore whether the intensity of happiness, anger, or sadness (either initially or at the time of retrieval) predicted the number of events recognised after a year. The predictors were identical to those entered in the regression analysis conducted on memory clarity after two months. No model significantly predicted event recognition. In summary, greater happiness about the verdict at the time of retrieval predicted greater memory clarity after two months, but did not predict event recognition after more than a year. This may have been because the intensity of participants' current feelings of happiness about the verdict faded considerably between two months and a year (see Levine & Bluck, in press).

Memory confidence after a year

Finally, we examined the relation between participants' emotional reactions to the verdict and their confidence in their memory judgements after a year. An

TABLE 4

Mean hit and false alarm rates, and measures of discriminability and bias, for participants whose initial emotional reaction to the verdict was positive, negative or neutral ($N = 87$)

Emotional reaction	*n*	*Hit rate* (*H*)	*False alarms* (*FA*)	*Discriminability* (D_L)	*Bias* (D_L)
Positive	20	.60	.55	.25	−.35
Negative	48	.49	.40	.51	.34
Neutral	19	.55	.42	.52	.17

ANCOVA was conducted on the mean confidence ratings for all recognition judgements for participants whose emotional reaction to the verdict was positive, negative or neutral. This analysis controlled for the number of correct recognition judgements as well as for prior knowledge and rehearsal. Memory confidence was greater for correct than for incorrect responses, $F(1, 84) = 6.16$, $MS_e = 0.83$, $p = .02$, but did not differ by valence, $F(2, 84) = 2.48$, $MS_e = 0.83$, $p = .09$, n.s. We also conducted a regression analysis to find out if emotional intensity predicted participants' mean confidence in their recognition judgements. The predictors were identical to those in the previous regression analyses except that the number of correct recognition responses was added as the first variable on Step 1. The results showed that greater confidence was predicted by greater accuracy, $t(84) = 2.07$, $p = .04$, ß = .22, and more rehearsal, $t(84) = 2.01$, $p = .05$, ß = .22, but initial and current emotional intensity were not significant predictors of memory confidence.[4]

DISCUSSION

The goal of this study was to investigate the relation between happiness and the malleability of memory for real world events. We assessed participants' memories for the televised announcement of the verdict in the murder trial of O. J. Simpson, using actual events and plausible foils. After two months, participants whose initial emotional reaction to the verdict announcement was positive recalled events with greater clarity than participants whose initial reaction was negative or neutral. Similarly, after more than a year, participants whose initial reaction was positive recognised more events than participants whose initial reaction was negative. This does not mean that those who felt happy about the verdict were more accurate, however—they were not. Happy participants recalled events with greater clarity, and recognised more events, independent of whether the events had actually occurred.

The intensity of happiness at the time of retrieval also played a role in how clearly participants reported remembering the verdict announcement. The happier participants felt about the verdict after two months, the more clearly they reported remembering events. Signal detection analyses, conducted on participants' recognition judgements after more than a year, showed that participants who were happy about the verdict used a more lenient threshold for judging that events had occurred than participants whose reaction to the verdict was negative. Participants who reacted negatively were more likely to err in a conservative

[4] The regression analyses reported in this paper were conducted on mean values for all events (i.e., mean memory clarity ratings, mean number of events recognised, mean confidence). We also conducted multivariate regression analyses with true and false events as the dependent variables. The results of these analyses also showed that greater intensity of happiness at the time of retrieval predicted greater memory clarity ratings after 2 months, and that emotional intensity did not predict recognition or confidence judgements after more than a year.

fashion by rejecting events. Thus, fewer errors of omission, and more errors of commission, were made when recalling positive events than when recalling negative events.

These findings are consistent with a growing body of laboratory research showing that people use different information-processing strategies when they are in a positive versus a negative mood. When making social judgements, happiness leads to greater reliance on general knowledge or schemas whereas a negative mood leads to conservative judgements that adhere more closely to the information presented (for reviews see Bless & Schwarz, 1999; Forgas, 2002). The differing information-processing strategies associated with positive and negative emotions have also been shown to affect memory. Inducing happiness leads to schema-consistent intrusion errors when remembering narratives (Bless et al., 1996) and to stereotype-consistent intrusion errors when recognising ethnic names (Park & Banaji, 2000). Closer to real-world events, in two eye-witness memory studies participants watched conflict scenarios. Later, they received a mood induction and were then exposed to misleading information. After intervals of an hour or a week, positive mood increased memory intrusion errors (unpublished studies cited in Forgas, 2002, p. 11).

The current study extends these findings to memory for real-world events that evoked happiness and to retention intervals of over a year. Memories become sketchy over time. Our findings suggest that people draw freely on general knowledge to reconstruct memories of happy events. Incorporating plausible or schema-congruent information from general knowledge when remembering events that evoked happiness would result in representations that are *experienced* as more complete. This may explain why people rate positive events as better remembered than negative events (e.g., Thompson et al., 1996), even though studies with objective measures often show no differences or even superior memory for negative events (e.g., Banaji & Hardin, 1994; Bluck & Li, 2001).

Memory for both negative and positive events become sketchy with time, however. Why would people report remembering more true and false aspects of an event that made them happy? Events that evoked negative emotions are goal-discrepant and indicate a problem to be resolved (Bluck & Alea, 2003; Levine & Safer, 2002). When remembering such events, people may engage in critical evaluation in the service of repairing past negative outcomes or avoiding future ones. In contrast, events that made people happy are consistent with their goals. Drawing flexibly on general knowledge when remembering such events may allow people to build on previous goal achievement without the risk that being slightly mistaken will lead to danger or difficulty (e.g., Fredrickson, 2001). Thus, when remembering happy occasions, people may "paint with broad strokes", remembering much of what happened but blurring the lines between actual and merely plausible events.

Examining "errors" in memory for real-world emotional events encourages us to re-evaluate what constitutes an error, and an error at what price (Bluck,

2003). The tendency to make errors can be weighed against the possible gain incurred from integrative information processing. ''Painting with broad strokes'' may be appropriate when remembering happy events. The same liberal tendency may be less prudent when negative events are recalled and lack of attention to details can lead to becoming embroiled in a new negative situation. As such, emotion may be an arbiter of how much risk of error is permissible in the pursuit of flexible and creative thinking.

Alternative explanations and limitations

An alternative explanation is that this is not a memory effect at all. Participants remembering events that made them happy may simply endorse positive (or higher) values on rating scales, including memory scales. If this were the case, though, happiness would have been associated with higher memory confidence ratings too, and it was not. Memory confidence, which is influenced by a variety of factors in addition to the subjective clarity or vividness of memory (Zakay, 1998), was not related to either emotional valence or intensity.

Another explanation is that participants might have used their emotions to inform memory judgements. When asked whether they remembered an event, participants may have asked themselves, ''How do I feel about it?''. and feelings of happiness may have been taken as indications of familiarity (Schwarz & Clore, 1983). The methods we used make this explanation unlikely, however. Research shows that when people's attention is drawn to the true cause of their mood, they typically discount mood, and it does not influence judgements (Gasper & Clore, 2000). In the current study, questions about participants' reactions to the verdict came before memory questions, making the source of their emotions explicit. Thus, the association between happiness and memory for both true and false information is most consistent with the view that happiness, at encoding and retrieval, promotes an information-processing style that allows the incorporation of reasonable but incorrect information from general knowledge.

Limitations of the study also should be noted. Because a quasi-experimental design was used, we cannot rule out the possibility that happy participants differed on some unmeasured factor from participants who had a negative reaction. Our confidence in the association found between happiness and memory malleability is increased by the fact that similar findings have been obtained in laboratory studies employing random assignment to positive and negative emotion-induction conditions (Bless et al., 1996; Park & Banaji, 2000). Also, although the verdict elicited intense emotion, future research is needed to confirm that the association between happiness and memory malleability extends to events with more personal consequences.

Conclusion

A pressing question in emotion and memory research is whether results obtained in brief laboratory studies generalise to real-world emotional experiences (Yuille

& Tollestrup, 1992). This study demonstrates that the association between happiness and reconstructive memory extends to memory for real-world events over retention intervals of more than a year. It supports a functional view of specific emotions: Happiness promotes flexible and constructive information processing not only in reasoning and judgement but in memory over time.

REFERENCES

Banaji, M. R., & Hardin, C. (1994). Affect and memory in retrospective reports. In N. Schwarz & S. Sudman (Eds.), *Autobiographical memory and the validity of retrospective reports* (pp. 71–86). New York: Springer.

Bless, H., Bohner, G., Schwarz, N., & Strack, F. (1990). Mood and persuasion: A cognitive response analysis. *Personality and Social Psychology Bulletin*, *16*, 331–345.

Bless, H., Clore, G. L., Schwarz, N., Golisano, V., Rabe, C., & Wolk, M. (1996). Mood and the use of scripts: Does a happy mood really lead to mindlessness? *Journal of Personality and Social Psychology*, *71*, 665–679.

Bless, H., & Schwarz, N. (1999). Sufficient and necessary conditions in dual process models: The case of mood and information processing. In S. Chaiken & Y. Trope (Eds.), *Dual process theories in social psychology* (pp. 423–440). New York: Guilford Press.

Bluck, S. (2003). Autobiographical memory: Exploring its functions in everyday life. *Memory*, *11*, 113–123.

Bluck, S., & Alea, N. (2003). Exploring the functions of autobiographical memory: Why do I remember the autumn? In J. D. Webster & B. K. Haight (Eds), *Critical advances in reminiscence: from theory to application* (pp. 61–75). New York: Springer.

Bluck, S., & Li, K. Z. H. (2001). Predicting memory completeness and accuracy: Emotion and exposure in repeated autobiographical recall. *Applied Cognitive Psychology*, *15*, 145–158.

Bodenhausen, G. V., Kramer, G. P., & Susser, K. (1994). Happiness and stereotypic thinking in social judgment. *Journal of Personality and Social Psychology*, *66*, 621–632.

Fiedler, K., Asbeck, J., & Nickel, S. (1991) Mood and reconstructive memory effects on social judgment. *Cognition and Emotion*, *5*, 363–378.

Forgas, J. P. (2002). Feeling and doing: Affective influences on interpersonal behavior. *Psychological Inquiry*, *13*, 1–28.

Fredrickson, B. L. (2001). The role of positive emotions in positive psychology: The broaden-and-build theory of positive emotions. *American Psychologist*, *56*, 218–226.

Gasper, K., & Clore, G. L. (2000). Do you have to pay attention to your feelings to be influenced by them? *Personality and Social Psychology Bulletin*, *26*, 698–711.

Holmes, D. S. (1970). Differential change in affective intensity and the forgetting of unpleasant experiences. *Journal of Personality and Social Psychology*, *3*, 234–239.

Isen, A. M., Daubman, K. A., & Nowicki, G. P. (1987). Positive affect facilitates creative problem solving. *Journal of Personality and Social Psychology*, *52*, 1122–1131.

Koriat, A., Goldsmith, M., & Pansky, A. (2000). Toward a psychology of memory accuracy. *Annual Review of Psychology*, *51*, 481–537.

Kreitler, H., & Kreitler, S. (1968). Unhappy memories of "the happy past": Studies in cognitive dissonance. *British Journal of Psychology*, *59*, 157–166.

Levine, L. J., & Bluck, S. (in press). How emotions fade: Valence, appraisals and the emotional impact of remembered events. *Advances in Psychological Research*. Hauppage, NY: Nova Science.

Levine, L. J., Prohaska, V., Burgess, S. L., Rice, J. A., & Laulhere, T. M. (2001). Remembering past emotions: The role of current appraisals. *Cognition and Emotion*, *15*, 393–417.

Levine, L. J., & Safer, M. A. (2002). Sources of bias in memory for emotions. *Current Directions in Psychological Science*, *11*, 169–173.

Mackie, D., & Worth, L. T. (1989). Processing deficits and the mediation of positive affect in persuasion. *Journal of Personality and Social Psychology*, *57*, 27–40.

Master, D., Lishman, W. A., & Smith, A. (1983). Speed of recall in relation to affective tone and intensity of experience. *Psychological Medicine*, *13*, 325–331.

Matlin, M. W., & Stang, D. J. (1978). *The Pollyanna principle: Selectivity in language, memory, and thought.* Cambridge, MA: Schenkman.

Park, J., & Banaji, M. R. (2000). Mood and heuristics: The influence of happy and sad states on sensitivity and bias in stereotyping. *Journal of Personality and Social Psychology*, *78*, 1005–1023.

Schwarz, N., & Clore, G. L. (1983). Mood, misattribution, and judgment of well-being: Informative and directive functions of affective states. *Journal of Personality and Social Psychology*, *45*, 513–523.

Snodgrass, J. G., & Corwin, J. (1988). Pragmatics of measuring recognition memory. *Journal of Experimental Psychology: General*, *117*, 34–50.

Thompson, C. P., Skowronski, J. J., Larsen, S. F., Betz, A. (1996). *Autobiographical memory: Remembering what and remembering when.* Mahwah, NJ: Erlbaum.

Walker, W. R., Skowronski, J. J., & Thompson, C. P. (2003). Life is pleasant—and memory helps to keep it that way! *Review of General Psychology*, *7*, 203–210.

Walker, W. R., Vogl, R. J., & Thompson, C. P. (1997). Autobiographical memory: Unpleasantness fades faster than pleasantness over time. *Applied Cognitive Psychology*, *11*, 399–413.

Yuille, J. C., & Tollestrup, P. A. (1992). A model of the diverse effects of emotion on eyewitness memory. In S.-A. Christianson (Ed.), *The handbook of emotion and memory* (pp. 201–215). Hillsdale, NJ: Erlbaum.

Zakay, D. (1998). Determinants of confidence in accuracy of knowledge retrieval. *European Journal of Cognitive Psychology*, *10*, 291–306.

COGNITION AND EMOTION, 2004, *18* (4), 575–585

Altering traumatic memory

Veronika Nourkova
Moscow State University, Russian Federation

Daniel M. Bernstein
University of Washington, Seattle, WA, USA

Elizabeth F. Loftus
University of California, Irvine, CA, USA

Can you experimentally contaminate memory for truly traumatic events? We investigated this question in a study in which 80 Russian participants reported on their memories for one of two terrorist bombings. Half the participants recalled the 1999 attacks on Moscow apartment buildings while the others recalled the 2001 attacks on the World Trade Center in New York. Participants recalled the events on two separate occasions over a six month period. Just prior to the second recall, we strongly suggested to all participants that they had seen a wounded animal in the attacks and had mentioned it in their original memory reports. While none of the WTC group were convinced by the suggestion, 12.5% of the Moscow group did so, and even elaborated with sensory detail (e.g., a bleeding cat lying in the dust). This group was more susceptible to contamination despite the greater emotion that they experienced about the Moscow terrorist attacks. These findings support the notion that even traumatic memories are experimentally malleable.

There has been substantial interest in the malleability of memory. Much work has shown that our memories can be altered, distorted, contaminated or even supplemented by new information that comes along at a later time. Naturally, as with most experimental studies of memory, the events in question are not particularly traumatic. This has prompted the question of whether highly emotional, even traumatic events in life, are similarly susceptible to such experimental alteration.

Brown and Kulik (1977) originally coined the term, ''flashbulb memory'' to refer to a specific type of memory that is a perfect and permanent mental

Correspondence should be addressed to Dr Daniel Bernstein, Dept of Psychology, University of Washington, Seattle, Washington, USA, 98195-1525; e-mail: db6@u.washington.edu

This research was supported in part by a Fulbright Fellowship to VN and an NIH individual National Research Service Award to DMB.

http://www.tandf.co.uk/journals/pp/02699931.html DOI:10.1080/02699930341000455

representation of an emotionally arousing event. Some writers have argued that traumatic memories are not readily susceptible to contamination, even taking the stronger position that such memories are immune to contamination. The claim is that they leave some sort of indelible fixation in the mind (e.g., ''traumatic events create lasting visual images ... burned-in visual impressions'', Terr, 1988, p. 103; ''memory imprints are indelible, they do not erase—a therapy that tries to alter them will be uneconomical'', Kantor, 1980, p. 163). In other words, proponents of this view would predict that experimental attempts to distort genuinely traumatic memory would fail.

There is anecdotal evidence that traumatic memories, like ordinary ones, are sometimes distorted. One frequently cited anecdote involves a highly public baseball tragedy (Anderson, 1990). Baseball aficionados may recall that Jack Hamilton, then a pitcher with the California Angels, hit the outfielder, Tony Conigliaro, in the face with a first-pitch fastball. Although Hamilton thought he remembered this horrible event perfectly, he misremembered it as occurring during a day game, when it was actually at night, and misremembered it in other critical ways.

There is other anecdotal evidence that very traumatic memories can be created in people. One of the most compelling such case resulted in litigation brought by a patient against her former therapist (Grumman, 1998; Holden, 1998). Patricia Burgus sued her former psychiatrist, Dr Bennett Braun for malpractice. According to news accounts and court records, Dr Braun used ''repressed memory therapy, including hypnosis'' (Holden, p. 6), which resulted in Burgus coming to believe that she was the high priestess of a Satanic cult. Moreover, she would come to remember such atrocities as eating thousands of babies in a year's time. Despite the absence of bones, missing person's reports, and any evidence, Burgus clung to these beliefs. Eventually, her lawsuit, also brought on behalf of her children, then aged 4 and 5 years, who had spent years in a psychiatric ward, brought a settlement that exceeded 10 million dollars.

One obvious problem with anecdotal evidence is that there usually is no way to verify the accuracy of the story (Loftus & Guyer, 2002a, 2000b). In the case of pitcher Hamilton, stories are told of his misremembering, but few have access to any ''original data''. In the case of Patricia Burgus, medical records and other evidence do suggest that she really adopted the false beliefs and memories, but there remains the possibility, however small, that she never truly held this bizarre set of beliefs. One other consideration in the typical anecdotal report is that the change in memory that is assumed to have occurred came about either spontaneously (as in the Hamilton example) or through therapeutic suggestion (as in the Burgus example). These did not involve a deliberate controlled experimental attempt to bring about that memory distortion.

There is also evidence of a less anecdotal, more experimental nature that supports the imperfections of personally experienced traumatic memories. The well-known study of people's recollections of how they heard the news of the

1986 explosion of the space shuttle *Challenger* is an example (Neisser & Harsch, 1992). Participants answered questions shortly after the explosion and again nearly three years later. More than one third were inaccurate. One participant, for example, learned the news from her best friend and later recalled learning it from television. A more recent study by Morgan and colleagues (2002) examined the memories of active duty military personnel who had gone through highly traumatic survival school training. Later many of them made errors when they tried to remember the individual who was primarily responsible for their torment. In both the Neisser and the Morgan studies, errors of traumatic memory were evident, but in neither study was there a deliberate experimental attempt to contaminate the traumatic memory.

There are a few important studies that did successfully use a leading question to plant a false suggestion into memory for a traumatic event (Crombag, Wagenaar, & van Koppen, 1996; Granhag, Stromwall, & Billings, 2002; Ost, Vrij, Costall, & Bull, 2002). In the Crombag et al. study, the traumatic event was the crash of an El Al Boeing 747 into an apartment building in Amsterdam, which occurred in October 1992. The plane crashed into an 11-story apartment building, killing the four crew members aboard the plane and 39 people inside the building. While no television crews filmed the actual crash, they did film the resultant fire and the rescue of survivors from the building. For several days this was the top news story, and virtually everyone in the country knew about it.

Ten months after the crash, the Dutch subjects were questioned about their memories, including a leading question that presumed that the moment of the crash had been shown on TV: ''Did you see the television film of the moment the plane hit the apartment building?'' If they responded in the affirmative, they answered follow-up questions such as whether they could remember how long it took for the fire to start. Of 107 respondents, more than half (55%) claimed to have seen the fire start. Of these, 59% said the fire started immediately upon impact, 23% said it took a little while, and only 18% said they could not remember. In a second study, an even larger proportion (66%) of respondents said they had seen a TV film of the crashing plane. Many reported highly specific memories (e.g., the plane was already burning when it crashed, that it hit the building horizontally, that it disintegrated after impact) that they could not have seen. The true facts were discussed in later news coverage: The fire actually started immediately, the plane crashed nose down and almost vertically, and the body of the plane fell to the ground. Of course, these facts could not have been personally witnessed, and if the subjects had taken the time to contemplate, they would have realised how improbable it was that the crash moment would have been captured on television. Nonetheless, this study documents the malleability of traumatic memories. Crombag et al. (1996) speculated that dramatic events may be even more vulnerable than ordinary events to post event influences, because they are often highly publicised and by their very nature may more readily evoke visualisation, thus interfering with our ''source monitoring'' capabilities. They did not manipulate the extent of trauma. Nor did they have an experimental manipulation that would have revealed whether it was the leading question that prompted the false recall, or whether it occurred through autosuggestion or some other process.

In more recent work, Ost et al. (2002) replicated the main findings of Crombag et al. (1996), this time using the Paris car crash that claimed Princess Diana's life. Nearly half (45%) of the British sample reported that they had seen a nonexistent film of the car crash.

In another recent study, Granhag et al. (2002) asked participants to read descriptions of film coverage of two disastrous events (the 1993 airplane crash at an air show in Stockholm and the 1994 sinking of the *Estonia*). There was actual film coverage of the air crash, but not of the sinking. The description of the nonexistent film of the *Estonia* was as follows:

> One night in September 1994, the ferry *Estonia* sank and over 850 people lost their lives. One of the marine helicopters came first to the scene of the accident. One of the rescue divers on the helicopter video-filmed the last pictures of the *Estonia*. On the short film, one can see how the ferry is standing almost vertically, prow up, and sinking slowly. Around the sinking ship, one can see a number of yellow rubber rescue boats drifting around in the rough sea.

After reading each of the film descriptions, participants answered questions about that event. Participants were told that each of the disasters was broadcast on television. They were later asked: ''Did you see the film?'' for each event. While 76% of participants claimed to have seen the actual film of the air crash, 38% claimed to have seen the nonexistent film of the *Estonia* sinking. In a second study, experimental and control participants were handed the same *Estonia* description and questionnaire as used in experiment 1. Experimental participants read the description and then overheard a confederate exclaim: ''*Estonia*—of course, I remember that film!'' (positive social influence) or ''*Estonia*—I can't remember such a film!'' (negative social influence). Control participants received no social influence. As expected, in the positive social influence, more participants claimed to have seen the nonexistent *Estonia* film (76%), than in the negative influence (36%). Controls were right in the middle (52%). These findings demonstrate the power of social influence in the formation of false memories for traumatic events.

Taken together, the Crombag et al. (1996) study and those of Ost et al. (2002) and Granhag et al. (2002) indicate that it is possible to convince people that they had seen footage of traumatic events that they could not possibly have seen. In some cases, this was accomplished by describing the film, while in other cases, the distortion appeared to be caused by a leading question that suggested the existence of such footage, for example: ''Have you seen the paparrazi's video-recording of the car crash in which Diana, Princess of Wales, and Dodi Fayed lost their lives?'' (Ost et al., 2002, p. 129). We say ''appeared to be caused'' because the question format was not experimentally manipulated, so no strong causal arguments can be made. We only know that distortions in memory for a traumatic public event do occur, and we know a bit about some factors that affect the degree of such distortion.

To our knowledge, only one study, an unpublished doctoral dissertation (Abhold, 1995) has demonstrated the experimentally induced malleability of memory for a serious life-and-death situation. High-school students had attended a football game at which a player on the field went into cardiac arrest. Attempts to resuscitate the player appeared to fail, and many students thought he had died (although he was later revived). Reactions ranged from complete silence, to sobbing and screaming. Six years later, many of these students were interviewed, and some were exposed to misleading information (blood on the player's jersey) about this traumatic event. More than a quarter of the students accepted the misinformation. This single study does show that experimental contamination of traumatic memory is possible. The delicacy of conducting such work (e.g., deliberate contamination of memories of those who have suffered) has probably been responsible for the dearth of additional research along these lines.

To address these issues and provide data to fill the aforementioned gap in the literature of memory malleability, we attempted to plant false information into memory for a truly traumatic event. We used a unique opportunity to examine memory for two different traumatic events that were personally and historically significant. The first critical event involved two separate terrorist bombings that occurred in two Moscow apartment buildings, one on 9 September 1999 (at midnight), and another on 13 September 1999 (at 5:05 am). The second critical event involved the terrorist attacks on the World Trade Center (8:45 am and 9:03 am) in New York City on 11 September 2001. The Moscow attacks claimed 233 lives, while the World Trade Center (WTC) attacks claimed nearly 3000 lives. We hypothesised that the two critical events would differ for the Russian sample used in this study. The Moscow attacks should be highly personally relevant to the Russian sample, but these same attacks were likely not of great historical significance. Conversely, the WTC bombings should be less personally significant to the Russian sample, but were likely of great historical importance.

We attempted to plant a false memory for having witnessed a wounded animal as part of the critical event. Such a manipulation could have one of four possible outcomes. Those who believe that truly traumatic memories are immune to such suggestive manipulation might predict that neither the group remembering the Moscow bombings nor the group remembering the WTC bombings would accept the suggestion. Those who believe that all memory is highly susceptible to strong suggestion might predict that both groups would fall sway to the suggestion.

There is also reason to predict that the Moscow bombings group would be less susceptible to suggestive contamination. If the event is much more personally significant, it might be more rehearsed, and it might be stronger, rendering it more resistant to alteration (Loftus, 1979/1996, pp. 130–131).

On the other hand, there is also reason to predict that the Moscow bombings group would be more susceptible to memory distortion. The critical event in question occurred much earlier in time (three years before the suggestive manipulation vs. one year before). Older memories have been found to be more susceptible to contamination (Loftus, Miller, & Burns, 1978), perhaps because they have diminished strength. Thus, it is possible that the older memory for the Moscow bombings would be weaker than that for the WTC disaster. As such, the older memory would be more prone to alteration.

METHOD

Participants

The participants were undergraduate students from Moscow State University in Moscow, Russia. In the first session, 91 individuals completed a questionnaire. In the second session, 80 returned to complete a new set of questions. These included 62 females and 18 males, with a mean age of 22.6, SD = 0.94.

Materials and procedure

Session 1 was conducted in March 2002, approximately 6 months after the World Trade Center bombings, and approximately 2.5 years after the Moscow bombings. During this session, participants filled out a questionnaire designed to induce them to recall and write about these tragedies.

Session 2 was conducted in late September and October, 2002, thus approximately a half year after Session 1. During Session 2, 40 participants were randomly assigned to answer questions about the WTC bombings (WTC Memory group), and 40 to answer about the Moscow bombings (Moscow Memory group). For their assigned event, they rated their memories using a 5-point scale that ranged from 1 (very low) to 5 (very high). They rated the event in terms of its personal significance, for example: ''How significant was the event to you personally?'' [translated from Russian]. They also rated the event in terms of historical importance, how emotional they were at the time of the event, and how emotional they are now about the event. These key ratings were embedded amongst a set of 12 items. Participants also described their emotional reaction to the critical event, in their own words.

The attempt to contaminate memory occurred in Session 2, and was accomplished by asking this question: ''A half year ago, when you were taking part in our study you mentioned a wounded animal. Do you remember it?'' They were asked to provide as much information as they could remember.

RESULTS

Ratings of WTC vs. Moscow

One possible outcome was that the Moscow memory would be less malleable because of its great personal significance for this sample. To check that our Russian participants did find this event to be of greater personal significance, we conducted *t*-tests comparing the two groups. Indeed, we found that the Moscow Memory participants rated the event as more personally significant than did the WTC Memory participants during both sessions: 2.95 vs. 1.85 for Session 1 $t(78) = 5.23$ and 3.48 vs. 1.5 for Session 2 $t(78) = 9.07$, $p < .01$ for both. By contrast, the Moscow Memory participants rated the event as less historically important during both sessions: 2.33 vs. 4.13 for Session 1 $t(78) = 9.75$ and 2.65 vs. 3.75 for Session 2 $t(78) = 5.78$, $p < .01$ for both.

In terms of emotional ratings, the Moscow Memory participants rated their emotions in the past as being stronger than did the WTC Memory Participants during both sessions: 4.25 vs. 3.65 for Session 1 $t(78) = 3.33$, $p < .01$ and 4.2 vs. 3.80 for Session 2 $t(78) = 2.54$, $p < .05$. They also rated their emotions now as being stronger during both sessions: 3.08 vs. 2.50 for Session 1 $t(78) = 2.56$, $p < .05$ and 3.50 vs. 2.38 for Session 2 $t(78) = 5.41$, $p < .01$.

To determine the consistency in ratings between the two sessions, we computed correlations between Session 1 and Session 2 ratings for each of our four variables of interest (personal significance; historical importance; emotions in the past; emotions now) for both the WTC and Moscow Memory Groups. The average intercorrelations were .18 for the Moscow Memory Group (Range = −.11 to .48) and .11 for the WTC Memory Group (Range = −.17 to .43). Thus, ratings during the two sessions were not very consistent for either group.

Not only did the Moscow Memory participants express stronger emotion, but they also characterised their emotions differently. Moscow Memory participants commonly expressed emotions, such as fear and empathy. WTC Memory participants commonly described the event using more cognitive terms, such as disbelief and astonishment.

So we did indeed find that the Moscow Memory participants regarded the event to be of greater personal significance, and one in which they experienced stronger emotions, both past and present. Would this make the event less prone to contamination?

(False) memory for a wounded animal

None of the participants in either group mentioned a wounded animal during Session 1. However, after receiving the strong suggestion that they had mentioned this detail, five Moscow Memory participants (12.5%) accepted the suggestion that they had seen and previously recalled a wounded animal during the Moscow bombings. In contrast, none of the WTC Memory participants accepted this suggestion ($\chi^2 = 5.0$, $p < .05$). While 12.5% is not large, it does show that it is possible with only a small suggestion to create aspects of memories for a traumatic event like the Moscow bombings. This small suggestion, however, failed to make anyone report a wounded animal at the WTC.

When describing the ''wounded animals'' three participants imbued the scene with elaborate sensory detail. One recalled an ''absolutely crazy dog, barking and rushing around police officers''. Two others described ''a lost parrot in a cage'', and ''a bleeding cat, lying in the dust''. A fourth recalled ''a broken glass, that could be a fragment of a home aquarium''. The final individual reported that he did indeed remember an animal, but his image was vague, and he gave no further details.

Who falsely remembers?

To gather further information about the five individuals who fell sway to the suggestion about a wounded animal, we separately calculated their ratings of personal significance and other aspects. We found that the ''wounded animal believers'' (i.e., false memory participants) rated the personal significance of the Moscow bombings as substantially lower than did those who resisted the suggestion (2.0 vs. 3.69) $t(38) = 3.64$, $p < .01$, despite the two groups being similar during Session 1 (3.2 vs. 2.9) $t(38) = 0.64$, $p > .1$. Moreover, they rated the historical importance as higher than did their non-misled counterparts (3.8 vs. 2.49) $t(38) = 3.50$, $p < .01$, despite the two groups being similar during Session 1 (2.8 vs. 2.26) $t(38) = 1.67$, $p > .10$. In terms of emotional ratings, the ''wounded animal believers'' and the ''resistors'' rated their past and present emotions similarly both during Session 1 and Session 2 (t-values all < 1.0).

Thus, the individuals who accepted the wounded animal misinformation and those who resisted the misinformation in the Moscow Memory group rated the personal and historical importance of the attack similarly during Session 1, but the two groups' ratings diverged during Session 2. Despite these rating differences during Session 2, the two groups had similar emotional ratings both during Session 1 and Session 2 (and both groups expressed greater emotion than did the WTC Memory group). So the particular set of participants who succumbed to the wounded animal suggestion happened to be a group that found the Moscow event to be less personally relevant, but still they were emotional about it. This contradicts the hypothesis that greater emotionality would protect the event from contamination.

DISCUSSION

We began this project with a simple question: Can you deliberately plant false details into truly traumatic memories? We attempted to convince participants that they had seen a wounded animal as part of their memory for a tragic bombing. We found a minority of participants fell sway to the suggestion and claimed to have seen a wounded animal, but only when we asked about the Moscow bombings, and not about the WTC bombings.

Our finding contradicts an often-asserted claim that traumatic memories are immune to such suggestive influences. Moreover, we showed that we could alter memory for an event about which participants reported strong emotion. The suggestion appears to have led to the planting of a false memory, and for some individuals one that is quite detailed.

One potential challenge to this claim is that perhaps this is not a false memory. Perhaps there were wounded animals around the Moscow collapsed building, and participants saw them even if they did not mention them in their time 1 reports. We regard this as unlikely. We checked Internet sites and television archives and found no evidence of wounded animals.

The greater malleability that occurred with the Moscow bombings fits with other research showing that older memories are more susceptible to contamination. The idea is that as a memory is weakened, there is less likelihood that people will notice a discrepancy between the suggestive information, and what they have readily available in memory. So the time factor could have contributed to the greater susceptibility we saw here in the Moscow Memory group (although see Kvavilashvili, Mirani, Schlagman, & Kornbrot, 2003).

There is at least one possible reason why only the Moscow Memory group accepted the suggestion and no participants in the WTC Memory group did. That is, we planted a suggestion about an animal. Animals are more likely to be seen in residential settings such as the setting for the Moscow bombings. Pets are far less likely to be seen in commercial settings. In that sense one could say it is rather implausible that animals would be seen, and some work on memory malleability indicates that it is easier to distort memory if the distorting information is plausible (Pezdek, Finger, & Hodge, 1997).

We acknowledge a drawback in our procedure. We chose the two critical events because they were both highly tragic terrorist attacks, and they happened to have both occurred in September, albeit separated by two years. For our Russian sample, the critical events differ in numerous ways. One is an older memory and more personally relevant. The other is more recent, and more historically important (see Smith, Bibi, & Sheard, 2003). One occurred in a residential setting where the planted false information was more plausible. The two events also differed in terms of the kind of post event media coverage that appeared. As is well known, there were television cameras at the WTC and images of the collapsing towers were widely disseminated. While 60% of Americans reported watching these events occur live on TV and over 99% watched some TV during the week following the attack (Silver, Holman, McIntosh, Poulin, & Gil-Rivas, 2002), it is unknown what the corresponding percentages are in Russia. We do know that some of the same ''live'' images of the WTC were repeatedly available. By contrast, there were no cameras at the

Moscow apartment bombings, so Russian citizens had only still images of the ruins to view in the aftermath. It would be ideal if in future research these various event differences could be minimised to help determine which factors are truly at the root of responsiveness to suggestive misinformation for a traumatic event.

Finally, it is worth noting that despite our ability to plant a false detail into a traumatic memory, we succeeded with only a minority of subjects. Thus, the vast majority resisted the suggestion, despite our attempt to convince them that they had even mentioned the detail earlier. While the WTC Memory group may have done so because of the low probability of the specific details that we suggested, this does not explain the wide resistance that occurred in the Moscow Memory group. This observation points to the need to develop theories of when people are vulnerable to such suggestions that contaminate autobiography and when they are resistant.

REFERENCES

Abhold, J. J. (1995). *The distortion of a distant and traumatic memory: Implications for eyewitness testimony and psychotherapy*. Unpublished doctoral dissertation. University of Arkansas.

Anderson, D. (1990, February 27). Handcuffed in history to Tony C. *New York Times*, p. B9.

Brown, R., & Kulik, J. (1977). Flashbulb memories. *Cognition*, *5*, 73–99.

Crombag, H. F. M., Wagenaar, W. A., & van Koppen, P. J. (1996). Crashing memories and the problem of ''source monitoring''. *Applied Cognitive Psychology*, *10*, 95–104.

Granhag, P. A., Stromwall, L. A., & Billings, J. F. (2002, September). *''I'll never forget the sinking ferry!'': How social influence makes false memories surface*. Paper presented at the 12th European Conference on Psychology and Law, September, Leuven, Belgium.

Grumman, C. (1998, September 24). More former patients come forward to assail psychiatrist. *Chicago Tribune*, p. NW 8.

Holden, M. W. (1998, October). Settlement survey. *Chicago Lawyer*, p. 6.

Kantor, D. (1980). Critical identity image. In J. K. Pearce & L. J. Friedman (Eds.), *Family therapy: Combining psychodynamic and family systems approaches* (pp. 137–167) New York: Grune & Stratton.

Kvavilashvili, L., Mirani, J., Schlagman, A., & Kornbrot, D.E. (2003). The effects of time delays and nationality on personal memories surrounding the death of Princess Diana and September 11. *Applied Cognitive Psychology*, *17*, 1017–1031.

Loftus, E. F. (1979/1996) *Eyewitness testimony*. Cambridge, MA: Harvard University Press. (Original work published 1979)

Loftus, E. F., & Guyer, M. (2002a). Who abused Jane Doe?: The hazards of the single case history: I. *Skeptical Inquirer*, *26*, 24–32.

Loftus, E. F., & Guyer, M. J. (2002b). Who abused Jane Doe?: II. *Skeptical Inquirer*, *26*, 37–40.

Loftus, E. F., Miller, D. G., & Burns, H. J. (1978). Semantic integration of verbal information into a visual memory. *Journal of Experimental Psychology: Human Learning and Memory*, *4*, 19–31.

Morgan, C. A., Hazlett, G., Doran, A., Hoyt, G., Thomas, P., Baranoski, M., & Southwick, S. M. (2002). *Accuracy of eyewitness memory for persons encountered during exposure to highly intense stress*. Unpublished manuscript, Department of Psychiatry, Yale University School of Medicine. (Presented at American Academy of Psychiatry and Law Annual meeting, Newport Beach, CA, 2002)

Neisser, U., & Harsch, N. (1992). Phantom flashbulbs: False recollections of hearing the news about *Challenger.* In E. Winograd & U. Neisser (Eds.), *Affect and accuracy in recall: Studies of ''flashblub'' memories* (pp. 9–31). New York: Cambridge University Press.

Ost, J., Vrij, A., Costall, A., & Bull, R. (2002). Crashing memories and reality monitoring: Distinguishing between perceptions, imaginations and ''false memories''. *Applied Cognitive Psychology*, *16*, 125–134.

Pezdek, K., Finger, K., & Hodge, D. (1997). Planting false childhood memories. *Psychological Science*, *8*, 437–441.

Silver, R. C., Holman, E. A., McIntosh, D. N., Poulin, M., & Gil-Rivas, V. (2002). Nationwide longitudinal study of psychological responses to September 11. *Journal of the American Medical Association*, *288*, 1235–1244.

Smith, M. C., Bibi, U., & Sheard, D. E. (2003). Evidence for the differential impact of time and emotion on personal and event memories for September 11, 2001. *Applied Cognitive Psychology*, *17*, 1047–1055.

Terr, L. (1988). What happens to early memories of trauma? A study of 20 children under age five at the time of documented traumatic events. *Journal of the American Academy of Child and Adolescent Psychiatry*, *27*, 96–104.

SUBJECT INDEX

Made in the USA
Monee, IL
13 September 2026

62976814R10083